INTERMITTENT FASTING FOR WOMEN OVER 50

Written by:
Judith E. Kelley

JUDITH E. KELLEY

© Copyright 2021 - All rights reserved.

The content contained within this book may not be reproduced, duplicated or transmitted without direct written permission from the author or the publisher.

Under no circumstances will any blame or legal responsibility be held against the publisher, or author, for any damages, reparation, or monetary loss due to the information contained within this book. Either directly or indirectly.

Legal Notice:

This book is copyright protected. This book is only for personal use. You cannot amend, distribute, sell, use, quote or paraphrase any part, or the content within this book, without the consent of the author or publisher.

Disclaimer Notice:

Please note the information contained within this document is for educational and entertainment purposes only. All effort has been executed to present accurate, up to date, and reliable, complete information. No warranties of any kind are declared or implied. Readers acknowledge that the author is not engaging in the rendering of legal, financial, medical or professional advice. The content within this book has been derived from various sources. Please consult a licensed professional before attempting any techniques outlined in this book.

By reading this document, the reader agrees that under no circumstances is the author responsible for any losses, direct or indirect, which are incurred as a result of the use of information contained within this document, including, but not limited to, errors, omissions, or inaccuracies.

JUDITH E. KELLEY

Table Of Contents

INTRODUCTION 8

CHAPTER 1: WHAT IS INTERMITTENT FASTING?...............................10

CHAPTER 2: HOW IT WORKS 16

    LOWERS INSULIN RESISTANCE 18

CHAPTER 3: BENEFITS 20

    IMPROVED MENTAL CONCENTRATION AND CLARITY.............................20
    IMPROVEMENT IN HORMONE PROFILE...20
    REDUCES INFLAMMATION 20
    SUPPORTS HEALTHY BODILY FUNCTIONS 20
    POLYCYSTIC OVARIAN SYNDROME AND INTERMITTENT FASTING............21
    METABOLIC RESET 21
    CHANGE IN CELL FUNCTION 21
    IMPROVED SLEEP 22
    MOOD AND MOTIVATION..22
    CARDIOVASCULAR HEALTH 22
    GUT HEALTH 22
    WEIGHT LOSS..23
    LOWER THE RISK OF DIABETES 23
    IT BOOSTS YOUR METABOLIC RATE 23
    CONVERT YOUR BODY FAT...23
    IMPROVE MUSCLE HEALTH 24
    BOOSTED ENERGY..24

CHAPTER 4: TYPES OF INTERMITTENT FASTING 26

    16:8 METHOD INTERMITTENT FASTING..26
    THE 5:2 METHOD OF INTERMITTENT FASTING 27
    ALTERNATE-DAY INTERMITTENT FASTING...28
    24-HOUR FAST/ONE MEAL A DAY 29
    EAT-STOP-EAT...29
    SPONTANEOUS MEAL SKIPPING..30

CHAPTER 5: GET STARTED/HOW TO PLAN? 32

    EATING WINDOW 32
    FASTING WINDOW 35
    ROUTINE...35

CHAPTER 6: WHAT TO EAT WHILE FASTING? 38

Foods to Eat for Women Above 50 During Intermittent Fasting 38
Foods to Avoid 40

CHAPTER 7: MEAL PLAN FOR 14 DAYS 42

CHAPTER 8: TIPS AND TRICKS 44

Practical Tips for Fasting 44
Cooking Tips 48

CHAPTER 9: COMMON MISTAKES 50

Rushing Into Intermittent Fasting 50
Expecting Intermittent Fasting to Change Your Life 51
Choosing the Wrong Fasting Plan for Yourself 51
Not Drinking Enough and Drinking the Wrong Stuff 52
Overeating When Fasting Ends 52
Eating Too Much in the Fasting Window 52
Forcing It on Your Self 53
Not Paying Attention to the Nutrient Quality of the Foods 53
Restricting the Food Intake Too Much 53

CHAPTER 10: INTERMITTENT FASTING AND EXERCISE 56

CHAPTER 11: BREAKFAST 60

Healthy Chia and Oats Smoothie 60
Cherry Almond and Cereal Smoothie 61
Banana Orange Smoothie 62
Crunchy Banana Yoghurt 63
Grapefruit Yogurt Parfait 64
Creamy Mango and Banana Overnight Oats 65
Bacon and Eggs With Tomatoes 66
Cinnamon Porridge 67

CHAPTER 12: LUNCH 68

Lemon Baked Salmon 68
Easy Blackened Shrimp 69
Grilled Shrimp Easy Seasoning 70
The Best Garlic Cilantro Salmon 71
Crispy Oven Roasted Salmon 72
Aromatic Dover Sole Fillets 73
Bacon-Wrapped Salmon 74
Japanese Fish Bone Broth 75
Ground Beef and Cauliflower Hash 76

CHAPTER 13: DINNER...78

GARLIC GHEE PAN-FRIED COD...78
THYME ROASTED SALMON...79
STEAM YOUR OWN LOBSTER 80
BACON WITH BRUSSELS SPROUTS AND EGGS..81
PAN-FRIED TILAPIA 82
BACON TACOS...83
CALAMARI RINGS..84
PINCHOS DE POLLO—MARINATED GRILLED CHICKEN KEBABS 85

CHAPTER 14: SNACKS 86

BLUEBERRIES BOWL...86
BACON AND CHICKEN GARLIC WRAP 87
COATED CAULIFLOWER HEAD 88
CAULIFLOWER CRUST PIZZA 89
CABBAGE CASSEROLE...90
SALMON WITH SALSA...91
ARTICHOKE PETALS BITES...92

CONCLUSION 94

JUDITH E. KELLEY

Introduction

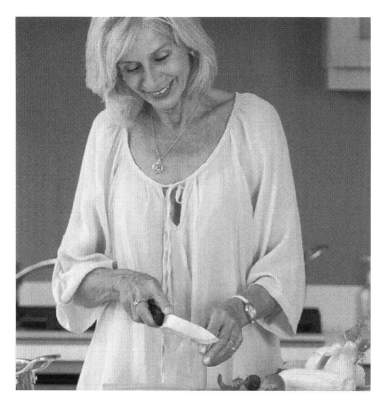

Intermittent fasting has become one of the most popular dieting strategies in recent years. It is been associated with everything from improving fertility to decreasing insulin resistance and the risk for some cancers.

There are many benefits of fasting for everyone; this book focuses on intermittent fasting for females over 50.

The goal of this book is to let women over 50 know about the benefits of IF, such as increased fat burning, reduced chronic disease, and blood pressure, improved insulin sensitivity, and other health improvements. Unfortunately, it seems like many women don't know about these fantastic benefits.

Women who practice IF usually start later in their life cycle: as a woman gets older, she might notice a change in her body composition. Her body composition is important because it can greatly affect her health. As studies have found, intermittent fasting may be a great way for women over 50 to lose weight.

If a woman over 50 wants their body composition to improve, she should exercise more frequently and eat healthier foods. A good time frame for eating would be an 8-hour window (one meal per day). Some people use this method simply for weight loss; they usually have one meal per day around 12–1:00 in the afternoon. The best time to eat starts around noon and ends in the evening. This is called the 12:12 window. The next best time frame is the 5:2 method; this means that women fast for 2 days out of the week and normally eat for 5. Another option is the 4:3 method; this means that a woman eats for 4 days out of 7 and fasts on 3. Although there are many ways to do intermittent fasting, these are 3 of the most common methods.

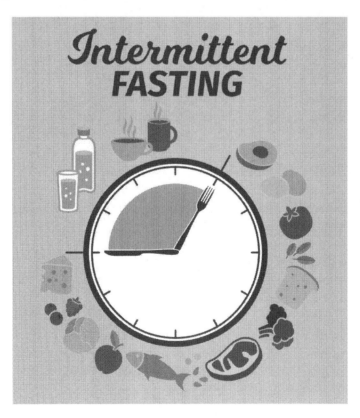

CHAPTER 1:

What Is Intermittent Fasting?

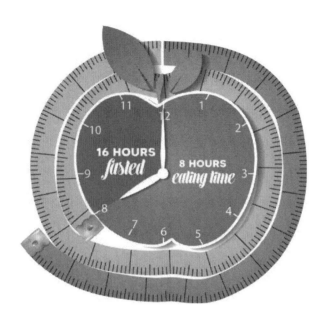

Intermittent fasting is the technique of scheduling your dishes for your body to obtain the most out of them. Rather than minimizing your calorie use by 50%, refuting yourself of all the foods you value, or diving right into a classy diet plan pattern, intermittent fasting is an all-natural, logical, as well as healthy, and balanced method of eating that advertises fat burning. There are tons of ways to approach intermittent fasting.

It is defined as an eating pattern. This technique focuses on altering when you take in instead of what you consume.

When you begin intermittent fasting, you will be more than likely to maintain your calorie intake the same; nonetheless, in contrast to spreading your dishes throughout the day, you will undoubtedly eat more significant recipes throughout a much shorter amount of time. As opposed to consuming 3–4 meals a day, you might eat 1 big meal at

11 a.m., afterward, an added large dish at 6 p.m., without any dine-in between 11 a.m. and 6 p.m., as well as also after 6 p.m., no meal up until 11 the following day. This is simply one strategy of recurring fasting, and likewise, others will be examined in this book in later stages.

Intermittent fasting is a technique used by whole lots of bodybuilders, specialist athletes, and also physical health and fitness masters to maintain their muscular tissue mass high and their body fat percent reduced. Recurring fasting can be done short-term or long-term, but the very best results originate from embracing this technique right into your everyday lifestyle.

The word "fasting" might stress the average person; intermittent fasting doesn't associate with starving yourself. To comprehend the principles behind effective intermittent fasting, we'll first look through the body's digestion state: the fed state and the fasting state.

For 3–5 hours after consuming a meal, your body remains in what is described as the "fed state." Throughout the fed state, your insulin levels rise to soak up and digest your meal. When your insulin levels get high, it is exceptionally tough for your body to shed fat. Insulin is a hormone produced by the pancreatic to handle sugar degrees in the bloodstream. Its purpose is to manage insulin; it is technically a hormonal storage agent. When insulin degrees come to be so high, your body starts shedding your food for energy instead of your conserved fat. This is why boosted degrees of it protect against weight reduction.

After the 3–5 hours are up, your body has finished refining the dish, and also you enter the post-absorptive state. The post-absorptive state lasts anywhere from 8–12 hours. Hereafter, when your body gets here, the time room is the fasted state as a result of the reality that your body has refined your food by this.

Factor, your insulin levels are reduced, making your kept fat extremely available for losing.

Persisting fasting allows your body to get to an innovative weight loss state that you would usually obtain with the average "3 meals daily" eating pattern. They are just altering the timing as well as the pattern of their food intake. It may take some time to get there when you start an intermittent fasting program right into the swing of points. Merely obtain back if you slip up right into your intermittent fasting pattern when you can.

Making a way of living adjustment entails a purposeful initiative, and no one expects you to do it completely today. Intermittent fasting will definitely take some getting used to if you are not in the practice of going long periods without eating. As long as you pick the right technique for you, continue to be focused, and also remain concentrated; you will unanimously grasp it quickly.

Unlike some of the other diet regimen strategies that you may embark on, the intermittent fast is one that will certainly work. When you hear about it, it is simple to be a bit terrified regarding fasting.

Recurring fasting is a little bit various than you might assume. If you end up being on, your body will often go right into hunger mode, rapid for as well lengthy.

You don't need to get as well concerned about exactly how this intermittent fast will work in the craving's mode. The intermittent fast is efficient because you are not going too quickly for as long that the body gets in right into this malnourishment setting as well as stops minimizing weight. Instead, it will make the fast continue long enough that you will have the ability to accelerate the metabolic process.

With the intermittent fast, you will discover that when you opt for a couple of hours without eating (usually no more than 2–4 hours); the body is not going to go right into the malnourishment setting. When complying with a recurring fasting plan, you require your body to melt more fat without placing any sort-of extra job.

Here are a couple of fast pointers for success:

- Mostly, it is essential not to expect to see outcomes from your new lifestyle promptly. Perhaps you need to focus on devoting yourself to the process for a minimum of 30 days before you can start to evaluate the results correctly.
- Second, it is imperative to remember that the excellent quality of the food you place into your body still matters as it will certainly merely take a few convenience food meals to reverse all of your tough work.
- For excellent results, you will plan to consist of an in-light exercise routine during fast days along with a far more fundamental regimen for full-calorie days.

Intermittent fasting describes nutritional consumption patterns that include not consuming or continuously limiting calories for a long-term period. There are various subgroups of regular fasting, each with variance in the duration of the fast of individuals, some for hours, others for a day. This has finished up being an extremely liked subject in the clinical research area as a result of every one of the prospective advantages of fitness in addition to health that is being found.

The diet regimen you adhere to whilst intermittent fasting will be figured out by the results that you are looking for and where you are beginning with additionally, so take a look at it on your own and ask the question, "what do I want from this?"

If you are looking to lose a significant quantity of weight, then you are most likely to have to take a look at your diet regimen plan extra closely, yet if you wish to shed a couple of pounds for the beach, then you could discover that a pair of weeks of intermittent fasting can do that for you.

There are many various ways you can do intermittent fasting. We just are most likely to consider the 24-hour fasting system in which is what I used to shed 27 pounds over a 2-month duration. You could really feel some cravings pains, but these will also pass; as you end up being even more familiar with intermittent fasting, you might find as you have that feeling of need no more existing inside you without concern. You might consider a juice made from celery, lime, broccoli, and also ginger, which will taste fantastic besides getting some sufficient nutrient fluid into your body. It would be best to stick to the coffee, water, and tea if you can handle it.

Whatever your diet strategy is, whether it is healthy or not, you should see a weight reduction after 3 weeks of intermittent fasting, as well as don't be put off if you don't find much advancement at first. It is not a race, and it is much far better to drop weight in a straight style over time, as opposed to losing a couple of extra pounds, which you will put right back on. After the initial month, you might want to have an appearance at your diet plan on non-fasting days and additionally remove high sugar foods and even any scrap that you might generally take in. I have discovered that intermittent fasting over the long-term tends to make me wish to consume healthier foods as an all-natural routine.

If you are practicing intermittent fasting for bodybuilding, then you may wish to consider having a look at your macro-nutrients and also working out just how much healthy protein and carbohydrate you call for to eat; this is a lot more complex, as well as you can uncover info about this on several websites which you will need to spend time examining for the very best end results.

There are great advantages to recurring fasting, which you will view as you proceed, a few of these advantages include even more energy, much less bloating, a clearer mind, and a basic feeling of wellness. It is important not to succumb to any type of lure to binge eat after a fasting duration, as this will negate the influence obtained from the recurring fasting period.

In conclusion, simply by adhering to a 2 times a week 24-hour intermittent fasting approach for a couple of weeks, you will slim down. However, if you can boost your diet plan on the days that you don't want to fast, then you will lose more weight, and if you can remain with this system, then you will certainly keep the weight off without turning to any kind of fad diet regimen or diet plans that are difficult to stick to.

JUDITH E. KELLEY

CHAPTER 2:

How It Works

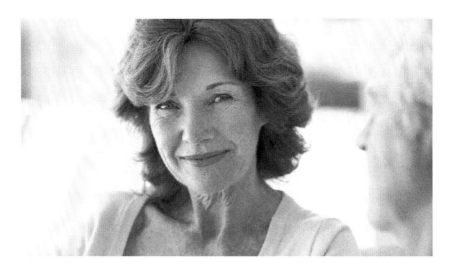

Intermittent fasting takes off the unwanted load from your internal system. It helps your body in regrouping its strength. Your vital organs get a chance to become more sensitive to responses. All this can happen by simply practicing extended fasting periods in your daily routine.

Excess of things is a major cause of problems in the body. We are keeping our bodies under the constant pressure of work. Eating and drinking may look like a fulfilling exercise but it is a task for the body to process the food. This task keeps the body engaged and doesn't allow it the time to relax. This leads to fatigue and various body functions start developing a kind of resistance.

To understand it in simple words you can take the analogy of cooking something in your kitchen. Let us suppose you have started boiling pasta. Pasta boils in a definite period of time. Neither overcooked pasta is good neither eating the uncooked one. Now suppose you start cooking pasta and add some more to the same water after 2 minutes.

You wait for 2 minutes and add some more. You keep adding more and more pasta after an interval of 2 minutes. In the end, you would be having a mess at your hand. Some of the pasta that was added in the beginning would get overcooked. Some of it would get cooked fairly while most of it would remain undercooked. You would have inedible pasta on your plate, although you boiled it for the desired period and followed the process thoroughly.

We are doing exactly the same with our bodies. Any specific meal, howsoever insignificant in quantity and light in nature takes a few hours to get digested properly. Experts believe that food takes at least 6–8 hours to pass through our stomach and the small intestine. From here the process gets very slow and the food gets absorbed very slowly. So, our body needs longer gaps between meals to process the food properly and absorb all the nutrients. However, we are not giving this time to our body and it is also causing most of the problems.

When we start our day in the morning we start with breakfast or an early morning snack this happens between 7–9 a.m. Between 11–12 people again have snacks and tea. This is a meal right before lunch which takes place between 1–3 p.m. The lunch causes lethargy in most people, and hence, tea and beverages come to the rescue. The evening snacks between 5–6 p.m. are also preferred by many people as this allows them late dinner and helps in eliminating hunger. The last meal of the day takes place ideally between 9–11 p.m. right before bedtime.

This whole routine doesn't give your body any time to relax. Your digestive system is always at work. It never gets those 6–8 hours to process a meal before the next one comes completely. You are simply adding more and more pasta to the same pot and spoiling the whole meal.

The food in our gut is not getting processed properly as our gut holds food items at various stages of processing that get the same treatment. This causes most of the digestive issues. Your body fails to absorb the required nutrients and you have no other option than to take nutrient supplements.

Your insulin levels always remain very high as frequent meals keep spiking blood glucose levels.

Your hunger and satiety hormones start responding in a wacky manner as the differentiation gets difficult.

You get prone to diabetes and insulin resistance in your body increases with time.

It also leads to an increase in your blood pressure and insulin resistance trips other vital parameters.

From chronic inflammation to the overactive release of stress hormones, the body is in a continuous struggle.

All this can happen simply because you choose to eat whenever you liked.

Now, think that you have been doing that for your whole life. When the body is in its teenage years, it has a very powerful digestive mechanism and there is a constant release of growth hormones. There is a high energy need, and hence, this doesn't affect us much and there is no significant weight gain. But once you cross teenage and start leading a bit sedentary life obesity starts kicking in. The digestive process starts getting weak and all the metabolic functions come under great strain.

The first thing intermittent fasting does is that it strengthens your digestive process by reducing the pressure from it. It gives your crucial functions like insulin formation the desired break and your system is able to relax. It is also the system that affects your fat storage, and hence, your fat-burning begins.

Intermittent fasting has a profound impact on most of your body functions and helps them in functioning better.

Lowers Insulin Resistance

What Is Insulin?

Insulin is one of the most important hormones in our body. It performs a very crucial function and that is to facilitate the absorption of energy by cells. Let us understand this in a simpler way.

Whenever you eat anything, that food gets processed and energy is released in the form of glucose. This glucose is released into the bloodstream and increases your blood sugar levels. Glucose is the simplest form of energy and all the cells in our body can use it directly for producing energy. This means that as soon as you eat or drink anything that contains calories your blood sugar levels rise.

However, there is a catch. Although your cells can use glucose directly for producing energy, they can't absorb it without outside help. You can consider the energy receptors to be locked which need a key for glucose to pass into the cells. Insulin is the key that can help in the process.

Our pancreas releases the insulin hormone as soon as it senses high blood sugar levels to stabilize the blood sugar level at the earliest. This insulin can bind itself with the cells and help in the absorption of energy.

A high blood sugar level is dangerous as it can lead to several health complications and persistent high blood sugar levels can also lead to multiple organ failure. If the blood sugar level remains high in general then it can also thicken the vessels in your vital organs and deteriorate their functioning. This is a reason people who have diabetes generally also have other issues like hypertension, heart problems, liver and kidney issues, chronic inflammation, etc.

CHAPTER 3:

Benefits

Improved Mental Concentration and Clarity

Fasting has incredible benefits for the healthy function of the brain. The most known benefit stems from the activation of autophagy, which is a cell cleansing process. Note that fasting has anti-seizure effects.

Improvement in Hormone Profile

There are plenty of people who avoid intermittent fasting as they feel it will cause their fitness levels to deteriorate. This is not necessarily the case for those people who do take part in intermittent fasting, as studies have shown that fasting doesn't negatively impact those who perform regular physical activities, especially if you cut down on your carbs as you fast and are in a ketosis state. Studies have shown that physical training while fasting can lead to higher metabolic adaptations.

Reduces Inflammation

Intermittent fasting promotes autophagy, a process in which the body destroys its old or damaged cells. Killing off old cells may sound like a terrible notion. However, it can be seen as a way of removing old and unwanted dirt from your body. It is a simple method for the body to clean and repair itself. Old and damaged cells can create inflammation. Because intermittent fasting stimulates autophagy, then it is possible to reduce inflammation in your body while fasting.

Supports Healthy Bodily Functions

Intermittent fasting gives your body time to complete processes and functions before introducing more food into your system. This means that every time you eat, you are giving your body adequate time to actually metabolize the food and use it appropriately. In modern society, we regularly overeat and push our bodies to be in a state of digesting constantly. As a result, our systems become overwhelmed and we don't effectively metabolize everything. This can lead to you not getting enough nutrition, storing fats, and struggling to produce healthy levels of natural hormones and chemicals within your body.

Polycystic Ovarian Syndrome and Intermittent Fasting

Polycystic ovaries are a fairly common disease in women. This disease causes a hormone shift and can have undesirable effects on women. Many women struggle with weight gain and difficulty losing weight as a side effect of the disease. While there are not very many studies about how intermittent fasting affects the disease, there is evidence that combining intermittent fasting with a Keto diet significantly helped to regulate the hormones and made weight loss possible for polycystic ovarian syndrome patients. There does seem to be some potential hope with using intermittent fasting to help treat and maintain diseases like polycystic ovarian syndrome and other hormonal disorders. Time and additional research will tell us if intermittent fasting has a future in helping with this disease.

Metabolic Reset

Many women, as they age, experience reduced metabolism. This is partly due to the natural aging process, and partly due to damaging the metabolism over the decades. Frequent crash dieting, poor sleep, overworking, poor health, and more can all damage your metabolism, thus preventing you from losing weight. But, by merely practicing intermittent fasting, you can reset and boost your metabolism, not only allowing you to lose weight but also helping you to feel healthier and maintain healthy lean muscle as you age.

Change in Cell Function

When you fast for a while, different changes take place in your body. For instance, your body will start a process of cellular repair and there will be changes in your hormone level. A difference in these levels makes it easier for the body to access the stored fat. You will notice that there is a reduction in the level of insulin and it helps increase the body's ability to burn fat. An increase in the human growth hormone helps to increase lean muscle and burn more fat than usual. Damaged cells are processed and other processes of cellular repair kick in. Also, several changes take place within the genes and molecules that protect you against disease.

Improved Sleep

There has been at least one scientific study that has shown that people who persist with intermittent fasting for 1 year or more have better sleep. The reasons why this occurs are no doubt complicated, but there have been conclusive demonstrations that intermittent fasting over an extended period assists in good sleep.

Mood and Motivation

The study of the effect of intermittent fasting on mood and motivation is in its infancy. There is a lack of research on large populations, using the statistical techniques of randomized controls. However, some studies have demonstrated that intermittent fasting does improve both mood and motivation in a surprisingly short period. As there is profound controversy about the pharmacological treatments of people's mental state, any treatment which has no side effects and many potential benefits must be considered seriously.

Cardiovascular Health

Intermittent fasting leads to a reduction in weight. For this and other reasons, it leads to an improvement in cardiovascular health. The cause of such disease is usually atherosclerosis, the deposit of plaque in blood vessel walls. The dysfunction of the endothelium, which is a thin lining of the blood vessels, causes atherosclerosis. A healthy endothelium works to prevent this insidious deposit. The endothelium is not doing its job properly if plaque builds up. Obesity, especially where the fat deposits are in the abdominal area, leads in many cases to this buildup of plaque.

Other causes of this deposit are stress and inflammation. Intermittent fasting assists in the reduction of these, as well as obesity. Some studies show improvements in all risk factors for cardiovascular health.

Gut Health

Increasingly, scientists are becoming ever more aware that microorganisms living in the human gut or digestive system perform vital functions. These are known as the microbiome. There are trillions of them and they are in other parts of the body, apart from the gut. Many diseases originate in the gut, not only illnesses concerning that part of the body, but also of the brain, the heart, and all other regions of the body.

There is research on mice that caloric restriction improves that part of the microbiome in the gut. The effect of this is to prolong the life of the mice. In humans, the effects of dietary changes are very swift, even as short as hours. Studies are currently being done to verify that the real effects of intermittent fasting observed in the gut health of mice are true for humans as well.

Weight Loss

The most obvious benefit of this diet is weight loss. When you follow intermittent fasting, the number of meals you eat will be reduced. When you eat less, the calories you consume will decrease as well. When the levels of insulin decline, growth hormone increases along with an increase in norepinephrine, which helps the body break down stored fat to provide energy. There is an increase in your metabolic rate when you fast, which helps the body burn more calories. The effect of intermittent fasting is 2-fold. On one hand, it increases your metabolic rate, and therefore, makes your body more efficient while burning fats. The reduction in the level of food you consume reduces your overall calorie intake.

Lower the Risk of Diabetes

The most common health problem that plagues humanity these days, apart from obesity, is diabetes. High blood sugar leads to insulin resistance in the body. Intermittent fasting helps to reduce blood sugar, and therefore, helps reduce insulin resistance in the body. When your body becomes resistant to insulin, it leads to an increase in the blood sugar level and the vicious cycle goes on and on. If you opt for this diet, you can successfully reverse this condition.

It Boosts Your Metabolic Rate

Studies show that staying in a fasted state leads to a spike in the hormone norepinephrine. This hormone increases your basal metabolic rate and burns fat. On top of that, once you enter your eating window, your metabolism still stays at an elevated level. You are essentially burning excess fat even when eating!

Convert Your Body Fat

Many people are unaware, but there are 2 types of body fat, white and brown. This fat is not created equal. Just as there is healthy and unhealthy cholesterol, there is also sturdy and unhealthy body fat. The white fat, which is what builds up as people gain excess weight, is damaging to health, contributes to aging, and leads to disease.

On the other hand, brown body fat is vital in protecting the body's inner organs and maintaining health. When you practice intermittent fasting, it not only helps you lose weight, but it can also actively convert your unhealthy white fat to healthy brown fat. As if that were not good enough, brown fat also helps burn off white fat, meaning that the browner fat you have, the more you will burn off excess white body fat.

Improve Muscle Health

Many people get excited about the temporary weight reduction they experience when trying the crash diet. That is until they stop losing weight and eventually give up on a diet. But, most of the weight loss people achieve on these diets is not fat loss but water weight and muscle weight. Muscle weighs more than fat, so even a small amount of muscle loss can make a big difference on the scale.

As crash diets promote malnutrition, it naturally leads to muscle loss, which negatively affects your health and strength as you age. After all, your muscles are in much more than your arms. They are surrounding your entire body, and even your heart is a muscle! As you lose muscle, your health and energy will be dramatically affected, and it is essential to regain this as you age if you want to improve your health. Thankfully, studies have found that when compared to dieting, intermittent fasting not only leads to more weight loss than dieting, but it also causes much less muscle loss. This means your muscles will become much healthier, especially if you actively workout while you practice fasting.

Boosted Energy

The mitochondria, which are within our mitochondrial cells, are the powerhouse of the cell. It is the mitochondria that allow us to use a variety of fuel sources from the food we eat as fuel, as well as ketones. While other cells in the body may only be able to utilize 1–2 fuel types for energy, the mitochondrial is incredibly versatile to be able to use all kinds of fuel. When you fast for longer periods (or are on a low-carb/Ketogenic diet), your body begins to produce ketones, which are then used to cross the blood-brain barrier and fuel the brain in the absence of glucose. But that is not all. When you are in this fasted state of ketosis, the body will also increase the number of mitochondrial cells within your body, replacing non-mitochondrial cells with mitochondrial cells, allowing for more of your cells to be fueled by any fuel source.

Since the mitochondrial fuel 90% of the human body, by increasing the number of these cells, you can naturally increase your energy. Not only will your physical energy increase, but your mental functioning and energy will, as well. This is great news for many people who lose energy as they age.

CHAPTER 4:

Types of Intermittent Fasting

All intermittent fasting methods are beneficial and effective, but it depends on the individual to find out which works better.

16:8 Method Intermittent Fasting

One of the most favored forms of fasting for losing weight is the 16:8 intermittent fasting plan. Often it is called time-restricted fasting, though some variants are subtly different. A person fasts for 16 hours in the 16:8 models and restricts the eating to an 8-hour window of time. As a portion of the 16-hour window, several individuals miss breakfast. So, for instance, you could eat during the 12–8 p.m. range.

Some people, though, choose to miss supper instead. You could restrict the eating window to 9 a.m. to 5 p.m. per day with this. To eat calories, a person can pick every 8-hour time and miss dinner or breakfast.

You might still eat the main meal a day for this fasting pattern. One can choose the timing of meals, like breakfast at 10:00 a.m.; lunch will be at 2:00 p.m., and dinner at 5:30 p.m. By 6:00 p.m., a person can finish eating their dinner so that all of the food consumption is done inside the 10 a.m. to 6 p.m. window, which is 8 hours.

The fasting limits the consumption of calorie-containing drinks and food to a limited window of 8 hours a day. For the rest of the 16 hours of each day, it involves refraining from food. Whereas other diet plans can set rigid rules and regulations, the 16:8 process is more flexible and based on the time-restricted feeding (TRF) method.

This fasting model may help one lose weight and lower the blood pressure by limiting the number of hours that one can eat throughout the day. A review study found that the 16:8 technique helped decrease body fat and maintained muscle mass in several participants when coupled with physical exercise. A much more recent study showed that the 16:8 method didn't hinder muscle gains in women performing aerobic exercise.

While the 16:8 technique can easily fit into every lifestyle, it may be difficult for some individuals to avoid eating 16 hours straight. Additionally, the potential benefits associated with 16:8 intermittent fasting can be negated by eating junk food or too many snacks during the 8-hour window. To maximize this intermittent fasting's health benefits, make sure to eat a healthy, balanced diet containing fresh vegetables, fruits, whole grains, good lean protein, and healthy fats.

The 5:2 Method of Intermittent Fasting

The 5:2 diet usually entails consuming normal amounts of calories to 5 days each week while reducing your calorie consumption for only 2 days of the week to 500–600 calories. Also known as the Fast Diet, this diet was popularized by British journalists. The 5:2 diet is a simple and direct intermittent fasting plan. You normally eat 5 days a week and don't limit your calories but also don't eat fried or unhealthy snacks. Then, you drop the calorie consumption to ¼ of your standard requirements for the remaining 2 days of the same week. This means reducing the calorie intake to just 500 calories each day, 2 days per week, for someone who regularly consumes 2,000 calories each day.

According to research, for people with type 2 diabetes, the 5:2 diet is as efficient as daily calorie reduction for weight loss and blood sugar control. Another study showed that the 5:2 diet for both weight reduction and the treatment of metabolic disorders such as cardiac failure and diabetes was almost as successful as constant calorie restriction.

As the person gets to select the days they are fasting, the 5:2 diet promises versatility, and there are no guidelines on whether or what to consume on full-calorie days. Having said that, it should be remembered that eating "usually" on full-calorie days doesn't grant you a free pass to consume anything you want.

It is not convenient to restrict oneself to only 500 calories a day, even though it is just 2 days a week. And, you can feel sick or faint from eating very few calories. The 5:2 diet might be efficient, but it is not for everybody. In order to see if the 5:2 diet could be appropriate for you, speak to the doctor. There are days for low calories, and you can eat around 25% of the calorie requirements, typically about 500–750 calories per day, and are sometimes referred to as "modified fasts."

It is recommended that women consume 500 calories on fasting days, and men consume 600. You can consume 2 regular meals of 250 calories per woman for 2 fasting days and 300 calories per man. No trials are evaluating the 5:2 diet itself, as opponents rightly point out, but there are loads of studies about the advantages of intermittent fasting.

- **Low carb group:** The 5:2 intermittent fasting has slightly larger decreases in insulin resistance and insulin relative to the low-calorie regular group. This category contained the most persons who had lost nearly 5% of their body weight.
- **Low carb group with fat and protein:** Intermittent fasting 5:2 lowered insulin and insulin resistance almost the same as the low-calorie regular group. This category has the lowest amount of weight reduction that came from fat. It makes sense as protein will try to stop fat burning (ketosis).

Furthermore, cholesterol levels, blood pressure, and inflammation were decreased for both classes. All intermittent fasting groups lost more body fat than the normal calorie restriction community. The investigators concluded that the IF 5:2 diet of fewer than 40 g. of carbohydrate a day produced the better outcomes of the 3 diets for body fat reduction and insulin sensitivity improvement.

Alternate-Day Intermittent Fasting

As the title suggests, every other day, alternate-day intermittent fasting is when one fast or severely limits their caloric intake. For alternate-day fasting, a person fasts every other day. The alternative fasting method every other day is much less popular. Furthermore, trying it is perhaps the most difficult form of intermittent fasting. This fasting routine may not be feasible. As per the review study, it may lead to intense hunger on fasting days. This other analysis revealed that most people who could do intermittent fasting were the respondents who tried to do alternative day fasting in an effort to lose weight. It also didn't generate greater weight loss or maintenance of weight. Usually, this intermittent fasting is not strongly recommended. For the whole day, it is difficult not to eat. The person should worry about their blood sugar, levels of insulin, and energy. Your ability to think can also be disturbed. You are going to be extremely hungry.

A professor of nutrition popularized this strategy. This fast consisting of 25 % of one's calorie needs almost 500 calories. On non-fasting days to be typical eating days, people could fast every other day. This is a common approach to weight loss. In reality, alternative day fasting has been seen to help obese people who want to lose excessive weight. By 2 weeks, the adverse effects (like extreme hunger) diminished, and by 4 weeks, the participants continued to become more comfortable with the diet. The drawback of that during the experiment's 8 weeks, respondents said they were never really felt their stomachs were full, which can make it difficult to adhere to this fasting method.

This intermittent fasting has several different versions. During intermittent fasting days, a few of them allow almost 500 calories. Some versions of this technique were used in many studies showing positive effects of intermittent fasting. A complete fast may seem far more extreme every other day, so it is not suggested for beginners. You can go to bed quite hungry several times a week with this method, which is not pleasant at all and, in the long term, probably unsustainable.

24- Hour Fast/One Meal a Day

Between meals, the trick is to fast for 24 hours. Eat at 7 p.m. on the first day, for example, and fast until 7 p.m. the following day. Conversely, a person can choose to eat earlier, either lunch or breakfast, and fast until the next day for 24 hours. The concept is that every day you eat a meal but allowing your body to fast for a longer period of time. This sort of fasting is usually performed once or twice a week, but it can be more frequently adopted. This type of fasting is not for everyone.

The OMAD intermittent fasting (one meal a day) is when one limits their eating window to only 1 hour per day, and for the remaining 23 hours, fasting happens. This is the ultimate type of intermittent fasting, and for many individuals, it can be an effective strategy for extreme weight loss.

Some of the risk factors of cardiovascular disease can be eased by this type of intermittent fasting but under strict medical supervision. During that window, one has to be able to last 23 hours without meals and resist the temptation to eat, as extreme hunger is a common complication of this sort of fasting.

Eat-Stop-Eat

Eat-Stop-Eat is an unorthodox approach to intermittent fasting popularized by an "Eat-Stop-Eat" journalist. This intermittent fasting plan includes classifying 1–2 non-consecutive days each week for a 24-hour cycle. During which one abstains from eating or fasting. One can eat freely during the remaining days of the week, but eating a well-rounded diet and avoiding overconsumption is suggested.

The reason behind a 24-hour fast every week is that eating fewer calories will ultimately lead to weight loss. Fasting for 24 hours can result in a metabolic shift that causes one's body to utilize stored fat rather than glucose as an energy source. But it requires a huge amount of self-discipline to avoid food for 24 hours on end and may lead to bingeing and excessive consumption later on. It may also result in eating disordered patterns.

In order to identify this pattern's potential health benefits and weight loss properties, much research is required regarding the Eat-Stop-Eat diet. Before attempting Eat-Stop-Eat, speak with the doctor and see if that could be an appropriate weight reduction solution for you. This strategy varies from other plans in that it emphasizes flexibility.

Spontaneous Meal Skipping

To enjoy any of its advantages, you don't need to adopt a formal intermittent fasting schedule. Another choice is to miss meals from time to time, such as cooking and eat and not consuming when you are too busy or don't feel hungry. It is a misconception that every few hours, people ought to consume calories before they enter hunger mode or lose their muscles. Your body is well prepared to cope with long stretches of hunger, let alone the loss of 1–2 meals from time to time.

Therefore, one day you just don't feel hungry, miss breakfast, and only have a good lunch or dinner. Or, if you are going anywhere and you can't seem to find something you want to consume, do it easily and momentarily. It is simply a random sporadic quick to miss 1–2 meals anytime you are tempted to do so. Only make sure during the other meals to consume nutritious foods.

JUDITH E. KELLEY

CHAPTER 5:

Get Started/How to Plan?

Intermittent fasting is one of the easiest lifestyles to follow. It has immense health benefits. Most people believe that for a thing to work, it has to be complex and difficult. That is not the case with intermittent fasting.

Maintaining strict eating and fasting windows is at the core of intermittent fasting.

Let us discuss them in some detail.

Eating Window

First, let us begin with the easier part. This is the window in which you are allowed to eat.

This book is especially for women over 50, but let us first discusses women in general. Food is very important for the hormonal balance of women. Prolonged food deprivation can cause hormonal imbalance. This is the reason women in their reproductive age are advised against strict calorie-restrictive diets or even fasting for very long periods.

There are studies conducted on mice that demonstrate that longer food deprivation of any kind for a consistent period can cause shrinkage in the reproductive organs. It can also affect hormonal secretion.

Therefore, young women should only practice only moderate intermittent fasting. Their fasts should not be longer than 14 hours. They should not even start with 14-hour fasts, to begin with. They should help their bodies adapt to the change slowly and gradually.

When it comes to women over 50, longer fasts can be performed without any restrictions as the risk of hormonal imbalances causing irregular periods or complications in conception and childbearing are not there.

Women over 50 have greater freedom in terms of the duration of fasts they want to undertake. This presents a very advantageous opportunity.

Women have a greater affinity to accumulate fat, but they are also more likely to shed the fat fast under the right conditions. Longer fasts help in beginning the process of ketosis, and hence, women can lose weight and burn fat much faster than men.

Hence, the hormonal conundrum that is a great problem for younger women doesn't pose much of a challenge to women over 50.

Women over 50 reaching their menopause get freedom from issues like menstruation. While this may be a great relief, other issues become more prominent.

For instance, problems like PCOS start troubling more where they should also have gone with their reproductive abilities. However, this doesn't happen.

Intermittent fasting with a correct diet can also help you in managing the symptoms of PCOS to a great extent. Frequent chills, mood swings, obesity, glucose tolerance issues, and other such problems would not arise if you practice intermittent fasting.

Getting back to eating, women over 50 can take the liberty of holding longer fasts safely as they get more accustomed to fasting. They are at a lower risk of health issues arising due to hormonal imbalances caused by food deprivation.

Eating Hours in the Fasting Window

While women younger than 50 are not advised to fast for longer than 14–16 hours, if you have crossed your 50s, you can safely take it a notch higher to 18 or even 20 hours if you feel like it.

However, in intermittent fasting, the number of calories you can eat holds very little importance, and the way and hours within which you eat them are way more important.

This means that your whole eating window, which spans from the time of the beginning of your fast until you finish the last meal of the day, is very important. This period is the eating window.

If you begin your breakfast at 7 in the morning and finish your last meal of the day by 5 in the evening, then you will have a 10-hour window.

Eating Discipline—Culling the Habit of Snacking

Another very important part of the eating window is following an eating discipline. You will have to improve the habit of eating.

We all eat mindlessly. We eat for the sake of eating. We don't mind having a few bites when invited to eat, although we may not be having any appetite or hunger.

We feel it comfortably fine to have a glass of cold-drink when offered by someone even when we are not hungry not realizing the fact that the glass of soft drink may have an equal number of calories as a full meal, and to top it all, they are empty calories which are even more dangerous.

We get tempted to eat when an intoxicating aroma of food passes through our nostrils. Our desire to eat goes up when we see sweets and desserts on display.

We like to eat when we are sad as there are foods that provide great comfort. It is a sad fact that in restaurants, there is a category of food categorized as comfort food.

We may only have 2 proper meals or less in 1 day but may have up to 10 incidents on average that may cause insulin spikes.

This is the habit of snacking that is causing the highest amount of damage to our system. Our digestive system gets crushed under a load of food, and it is unable to process that much food. This leads to the passing of most nutrients through the stool unabsorbed.

It also causes irreparable damage to our insulin system, causing insulin resistance. It overloads your whole pancreatic system making it overwork and the beta cells may lose the ability to produce the required amount of insulin in the future; this problem is known as diabetes.

The most important step towards following eating discipline is to stop eating indiscriminately. You will have to put an end to the habit of snacking. This is a habit that is only taking you towards a health doom. You can only have 2–3 nutrient-dense meals in a day that can help in providing nutrition and energy.

Too many women fail at this; this can sound intimidating, but it comes very naturally with practice.

You will have to begin by lowering the number of snacks you have in a day and then bring it to a minimum.

You will also have to eliminate sweets and refined carbs from your diet as they lead to food cravings. The sweeter you will have in your diet, the faster you will feel more inclined to eat. If you have more fat and protein in your diet, you will feel less inclined to eat as our gut takes much longer to process them, and they keep releasing energy at a steady rate for much longer.

This is the basic preparation before you begin intermittent fasting. You must remember that intermittent fasting is not some magical formula;

it is a way to discipline the body to perform in an ideal way. This can't happen if you practice intermittent fasting but don't stop having snacks at short intervals in your eating windows. This would keep causing insulin spikes and your system would remain under duress.

Another thing with snacks is that they are mostly made up of refined flour and sweets. This makes them addictive, and you have stronger cravings for them. There are not snacks rich in fat and protein as they would become proper meals then and you are less likely to feel inclined to eat after having them.

Therefore, eliminate snacks from your life, and you will be able to get the benefits of intermittent fasting.

Fasting Window

Fasting windows are much simpler. There are very few restrictions in place apart from the eating ban. You can't eat in your fasting window is a comprehensive term, and it also includes consumption of calories even through drinking.

You are allowed to drink water, and it is very helpful to drink plenty of water as and when you feel thirsty. This will help your body in flushing out the toxins during the initial cleaning phase. But besides water, there are very few things that you can safely consume.

You can't drink any kind of sweetened beverage. You can't consume anything that has calories, even a few. This leaves out all kinds of sweetened soft drinks, alcoholic beverages, fruits, and other such things. There needs to be a complete blanket ban on the consumption of calories in any form.

For women, in general, the fasting windows can range anywhere between 14–16 hours. However, if you are a woman over 50 and you have been practicing intermittent fasting for quite some time, you can experiment with longer fasts as long as you feel comfortable.

There is only one simple rule when you get accustomed to longer fasts, and that is not to overdo things. Try to maintain a routine.

Routine

It is a very important topic that seldom gets any limelight in weight loss, but it is equally important, like everything else. If you don't follow a routine, you will find it increasingly difficult to follow a fasting schedule.

Have you ever noticed that some people eat very less or after very long intervals, and they don't feel hungry while you may find it hard to stay away from food even for short intervals?

This happens because our hunger system works like clockwork.

Another interesting fact is that hunger pangs are temporary. This means that if you stop paying attention to these hunger pangs and divert your attention to something else, you may not feel the hunger pangs after some time. This happens because the ghrelin release is limited.

This is important to understand because shifting your fasting timings can have a toll on your tolerance.

For instance, if you start beginning your fasts around 6 in the evening and break your fasts at 10 in the morning, after a few days, your ghrelin release would get timed accordingly. This means that you will start having strong hunger pangs in the morning at around 10 and around 6 in the evening to facilitate the intake of food. This would also mean that you will feel less inclined to eat during your fasting window.

However, if you follow an erratic fasting routine in which you begin your fast one day at 4 in the evening, 6 on another day, and at 8 on yet another day, your ghrelin release would never be able to time itself, and you will have to see longer periods of hunger pangs.

You will have frequent gastric juice release in your system when there is no food to digest and that can also cause problems like flatulence, and acid reflux.

Therefore, it is very important that you follow a fixed routine in your fasting schedule and don't change the timings very often. This will help you in practicing fasting in a much easier way.

JUDITH E. KELLEY

CHAPTER 6:

What to Eat While Fasting?

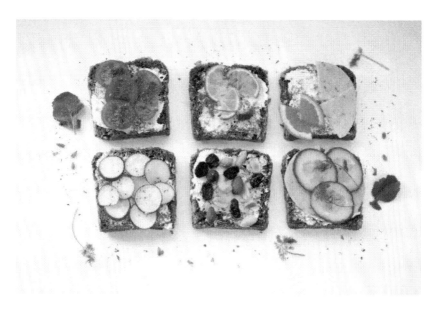

Foods to Eat for Women Above 50 During Intermittent Fasting

The dietary needs of a 50 years old woman are very different from that of younger females. Your body requires slightly different foods and nutrition than those of teenage females and even middle-aged women. Therefore, you will need to know what works and what doesn't. At this age, your metabolism is not going to be as efficient as before. You will know that by the changes your body is going through. Some foods will have a reaction they never had before. Similarly, your bones are going to lose their density. Your bones will become weaker than before. It is quite likely that no one diet is going to be efficient for you. However, a healthy meal plan and the pattern are going to do wonders for you.

Given below are the kinds of food types you need as a woman above 50.

Foods That Satisfy Daily Calorie Needs

Your body processes calories are slower than before. This is in a direct link to a slower metabolism. Since calories are going to be burned slower than before, you are going to need fewer calories. This is because when you were younger, you would have needed more calories since your body was growing. However, at this stage, your body has reached a certain stage. It processes things slowly, and calories are one of them. Therefore, you don't need as much as you did once you were 30 or 20. You need about 1,800 calories to maintain your weight. Some women eat less than before. However, some also overeat, which is not a good habit. You should be eating foods that satisfy your calorie requirements, taste good, and are nutrient-dense. Some of these foods are:

- Vegetables
- Fresh fruits
- Lean meats
- Fish
- Beans and legumes
- Nuts and seeds
- Eggs
- Dairy

Foods That Support Hormone Changes

I will not lie. Menopause is hell, and the hormone changes that you experience can easily throw you off balance. There are many side effects, such as night sweats, hot flashes, unpredictable mood swings, etc. These are usually symptoms of pre-menopause and post-menopause. When you do intermittent fasting after menopause, make sure to include all of these food groups. The first thing you can do that promises good hormone changes is an omega-3 fatty acid. These particular nutrients can be found in cold-water fish like salmon, sardines, and tuna. Flax seeds are also among the foods that can provide a natural supply. Flaxseeds also supply a type of fiber that is helpful during hot flashes. You may also want to consider foods that come from soy such as soymilk and tofu that ease menopausal symptoms.

Foods for Bone Health

Women over 50 need to be careful about bone health as the bones become less dense, and they start lacking in nutrients. This makes the bones weaker than before. As such, a diet rich in vitamin D and calcium is generally preferred. You will find that yogurt, cow's milk, goat's milk, cheese, and similar foods are usually a big yes for you. Many vegetables are rich in calcium. You will end up needing all of them. Generally, your main goal is getting vitamin D, and sunlight will provide you that. Getting more sunlight is the best way to get vitamin D naturally. You may also take vitamin D supplements. However, make sure before you start anything to consult with your doctor.

Antioxidants Foods

You need foods that will help you ward off free radicals. These are rogue molecules that are formed as you age towards your 50s. The free radicals' molecules damage cells and decrease your immunity. The immunity, if diminished, will make you more vulnerable to diseases. Consequently, you should be eating foods with a high content of vitamin C such as all citrus fruits.

Foods to Avoid

You often hear health experts demonizing sugar and carbs. Now, it should be said that sugar and carbs are not necessarily bad. They become a problem when they are consumed in excess. When you eat too many of these foods, your body has to play catch-up. Naturally, this is where you accumulate fat, gain weight, and see the adverse effects of an unhealthy diet.

So, the intermittent fasting approach calls for you to avoid, or at least significantly reduce, the following foods:

White Starchy Foods

This includes past and potatoes. Starch is metabolized as glucose and immediately goes into fat stores.

Foods Loaded With Carbs

White bread, or anything baked, is usually loaded with a high amount of carbs.

Greasy Foods

Deep-fried and very greasy foods, while tasty, are high in unhealthy fats. These types of fats lead to high cholesterol. These foods are enemy number one for blood vessel health. They generally lead to poor circulation.

Salty Foods

There is nothing wrong with salt unless you eat too much of it. Salting foods to taste is fine. However, excessively salty foods are not only addictive, but they affect your blood pressure and heart health. It is best to switch to sea salt as it contains less sodium.

Sugary Drinks and Alcohol

By "sugary," we mean things like sodas and iced teas. These are loaded with sugar and other chemicals. Also, alcoholic beverages end up accumulating fat in a heartbeat. Now, consuming moderate amounts of alcohol is perfectly fine (1–2 drinks per week). In fact, a glass of wine will be great for your heart. However, excessive alcohol consumption leads to increased fat gains. The reasoning behind this is that alcohol is metabolized by the body the same way sugar is. So, this implies you will be packing extra glucose into your system.

Also, check with your doctor to see if you have any unknown food allergies. Unfortunately, many folks out there go through their entire lives not knowing they are, in fact, allergic to certain foods. For instance, some folks are lactose intolerant but don't know it. Other common food allergies are gluten and corn. In particular, corn allergies can lead to quite a bit of digestive distress and inflammation. This is important to note as many of the foods we consume have corn in them.

CHAPTER 7:

Meal Plan for 14 Days

DAY	BREAKFAST	LUNCH	DINNER	SNACKS
1	Healthy chia and oats smoothie	Lemon baked salmon	Garlic ghee pan-fried cod	Blueberries bowl
2	Cherry almond and cereal smoothie	Easy blackened shrimp	Thyme roasted salmon	Bacon and chicken garlic wrap
3	Banana orange smoothie	Grilled shrimp easy seasoning	Steam your own lobster	Coated cauliflower head
4	Crunchy banana yogurt	The best garlic cilantro salmon	Bacon with Brussels sprouts and eggs	Cauliflower crust pizza
5	Grapefruit yogurt parfait	Crispy oven-roasted salmon	Pan-fried tilapia	Cabbage casserole
6	Creamy mango and banana overnight oats	Aromatic Dover sole fillets	Bacon tacos	Salmon with salsa
7	Bacon and eggs with tomatoes	Bacon-wrapped salmon	Calamari rings	Artichoke petals bites
8	Cinnamon porridge	Japanese fish bone broth	Pinchos de pollo—Marinated grilled chicken kebabs	Eggplant fries

9	Cinnamon and pecan porridge	Ground beef and cauliflower hash	Chicken and prosciutto spiedini	Parmesan crisps
10	Sesame-seared salmon	Cheesy taco skillet	Slow cooker bacon and chicken	Roasted broccoli
11	Eggs and salsa	Zoodle soup with Italian meatballs	Garlic bacon wrapped chicken bites	Cheesy crackers
12	Poached egg	Mini Thai lamb salad bites	Smokey bacon chicken meatballs	Almond bark
13	Creamy raspberry cheesecake bites	Bacon egg and sausage cups	Asian chicken wings	Coconut chocolate chip cookies
14	Decadent cherry chocolate almond clusters	Smoked salmon and avocado stacks	Baked garlic ghee chicken breast	Cheesy tuna pasta

CHAPTER 8:

Tips and Tricks

Practical Tips for Fasting

Practice indeed makes perfect. To help you get in the intermittent fasting, I have outlined a few down-to-earth routes and hands-on tips to guide you. Your approach to fasting can mean the difference between success and failure. So, consider these tips as guidelines that will help safely implement your preferred fasting regimen.

Find a Worthy Goal

First things first: Find a goal that is worth pursuing, or else you will drop the idea at the first sign of resistance. If you don't have a goal that represents a strong ideal, it will not be long before you start telling yourself, "I think I have passed the stage of such childishness." And yes, many women start a new lifestyle change for reasons that they can't keep up when things get tough. For example, the desire to look like models on TV, or social media makes losing weight feel socially acceptable and ok to keep up with trends that can be harmful. These reasons are not enough to keep anyone committed to a full lifestyle change and few wonder why so many people with goals are quick to jump from one lifestyle to another.

Don't go into fasting intermittently because it is the thing to do at the moment. Instead, look for inspiring goals such as:

- Staying fit, young, and healthy.
- Improving your cognitive or brain functions.
- Improving your overall vitality and increase energy levels.
- Balancing hormones, especially during menopausal or post-menopausal stages of life.
- Improving your overall health, thereby increasing longevity.

Do any of these sound good to you? Surely at this stage of your life, you are aware of the inherent risks of doing something merely because others are doing it too. That type of motivation will fail you.

Check Your Hormones

A woman's hormones can be easily thrown out of whack by the slightest change in her already established pattern of behavior. Whether it is a physical change such as altering your eating pattern or an emotional change such as being irritated or sad, it can bring about hormonal imbalance in a woman even if it is temporary.

But for perimenopausal and menopausal women, hormones can go haywire for reasons even they can't define. She could be feeling really great all week, and without anything changing she could suddenly become fatigued, depressed, and not in the right frame of mind. These changes happen due to the unpredictability of this phase of a woman's life. Because this can happen for no apparent reason, it is best to check your hormonal levels before putting your body through a major lifestyle change. If you have ever had issues with thyroid, cortisol, or adrenal fatigue, ensures that you have these checks before you begin.

This may come as a surprise to some women, but your ovaries produce testosterone too. So, as you grow older and begin to experience a decline in your estrogen and progesterone levels, your testosterone levels are also taking a nosedive. Your libido can be affected by low levels of testosterone and make you feel exhausted and bummed-out for no reason at all. So, while you are checking your other hormones, don't forget to do a testosterone test. The thyroid and testosterone hormones also help in weight regulation. So, if you intend to shed some weight using intermittent fasting, these tests are very necessary.

Start Slow

To go from having 5–6 meals daily to eating only once a day can lead to very dire consequences. In addition to being harmful to your health, massive abrupt changes are hardly sustainable. After confirming that intermittent fasting is suitable for your health, the next thing to do is planning how to ease into the habit. Before you fully implement any intermittent fasting regimen, it is a good practice to first test the waters, so to speak, with a less strict form of fasting. By doing this, it will help your body acclimate to the changes before going into the proper regimen.

Don't Fuss Over What You Can Eat

One common mistake people make when fasting is obsessing over the fasting hours and what to eat when they are finally allowed. You don't have to worry about if you are fasting as long as someone else, the important thing is what is comfortable for you. Of course, if your fasting window is too small, you are not likely to see any result. Also, don't get too tied up in every little detail of intermittent fasting. For example, you don't have to become too worried because you missed a day. Remember that fasting intermittently should be a lifestyle change if you want to continue to reap the benefits. And for a lifestyle change to be sustainable, you must be able to adapt and use it in a way that even if you face challenges, you will work your way around it somehow. Missing a day or cutting your fast short for reasons beyond your control should not get you worked up and worrying about whether you can do the entire plan. Don't give up.

Again, some people focus too much on what they can eat or not eat. For example, "Can I add just a little butter or cream?" "Would it hurt to eat this type of food during the fasting window?" If your focus is on what you can have or eat while you are fasting, you are giving your attention to the wrong things and putting your mind in an unhelpful state. Give your mind the right focus by concentrating on doing a good, clean, fast, and try to consume only water, tea, or coffee during the window.

Watch Electrolytes

Your body electrolytes are compounds and elements that occur naturally in body fluids, blood, and urine. They can also be ingested through drinks, foods, and supplements. Some of them include magnesium, calcium, potassium, chloride, phosphate, and sodium. Their functions include fluid balance, regulation of the heart and neurological function, acid-base balance, oxygen delivery, and many other functions.

It is important to keep these electrolytes in a state of balance. But many people who practice fasting tend to neglect this and run into problems. Here is a common notion: "Don't let anything into your stomach until the end of your fast" Even those just starting, know fasting doesn't work that way, and they tend to forget or fully stay away from liquids during their fasting window.

When you lose too much water from your body through sweating, vomiting, and diarrhea, or you don't have enough water in your body because you don't drink enough liquids, you increase the risk of electrolyte disorders. It is not okay to drink tea or black coffee throughout the morning period of your fast window. You will wear yourself down if you don't drink enough water. The longer you fast without water, the higher your chances of flushing out electrolytes and running into trouble. You can end up raising your blood pressure; develop muscle twitching and spasms, fatigue, fast heart rate or irregular heartbeat, and many other health problems.

On the other hand, drinking too much water can also tip the water-electrolyte balance. What you want to do is to drink adequate amounts of water and not excess water, whether you are fasting or not.

Give the Calorie Restriction a Rest

Remember that intermittent fasting is different from dieting. Your focus should be on eating healthily during your eating window or eating days instead of focusing on calorie restriction. Even if you are fasting for weight loss, don't obsess over calories. Following a fasting regimen is enough to take care of the calories you consume. It is absolutely unnecessary to engage in a practice that can hurt your metabolism. Combining intermittent fasting with eating too little food in your eating window because you are worried about your calorie intake can cause problems for your metabolism.

One of the major reasons that people push themselves into restricting calories while fasting is their concern for rapid weight loss. You need to be wary of any process that brings about drastic physical changes to your body in very short amounts of time. While it is okay to desire quick results, your health and safety are more important. When you obsess or worry that you are not losing weight as quickly as you want, you are not helping matters. Instead, you are increasing your stress level, and that is counterproductive. You are already taking practical steps toward losing weight by intermittent fasting, why would you want to undo your hard work by unnecessary worrying?

Simply focus on following a sustainable intermittent fasting regimen and let go of the need to restrict your calorie intake. Intermittent fasting will give your body the right number of calories it needs if you do it properly.

The First Meal of the Eating Window Is Key

Breaking your fast is a crucial part of the process because if you don't get it right, it could quickly develop into unhealthy eating patterns. When you break your fast, it is important to have healthy foods around to prevent grabbing unhealthy feel-good snacks. Make sure what you are eating in your window is not a high-sugar or high-carb meal. I recommend that you consider breaking your fast with something that is highly nutrient-dense such as a green smoothie, protein shake, or healthy salad.

As much as possible, avoid breaking your fast with foods from a fast-food restaurant. Eating junk foods after your fast is a quick way to ruin all the hard work you have put in during your fasting window. If, for any reason, you can't prepare your meal, ensure that you order very specific foods that will complement your effort and not destroy what you have built.

Break Your Fast Gently

It is okay to feel very hungry after going for a long time without food, even if you were drinking water all through the fasting window. This is particularly true for people who are just starting with fasting. But don't let the intensity of your hunger push you to eat. You don't want to force food hurriedly into your stomach after going long without food, or you might hurt yourself and experience stomach distress. Take it slow when you break your fast. Eat light meals in small portions first when you break your fast. Wait for a couple of minutes for your stomach to get used to the presence of food again before continuing with a normal-sized meal. The waiting period will douse any hunger pangs and remove the urge to rush your meal. For example, break your fast with a small serving of salad and wait for about 15 minutes. Drink some water and then, after about 5 more minutes, you can eat a normal-sized meal.

Cooking Tips

1. **Increase the amount of low-calorie.** Green vegetables are difficult to eat and should be purchased a bit earlier if large quantities are needed. Stir-fried vegetables are delicious. It is best to steam lightly. Invest in a tiered bamboo steamer to promote health and cook protein and vegetables at various stages that are environmentally friendly.

2. **Some vegetables will benefit from cooking, but other vegetables should be eaten raw.** Cooking certain vegetables, such as carrots, spinach, mushrooms, asparagus, cabbage, and peppers, destroys cell structure without destroying vitamins, allowing them to absorb more food. Mandolin makes the preparation of raw vegetables quick and easy.

3. **Fasting days should be low in fat and not fat-free.** A teaspoon of olive oil can be used for cooking or sprinkled on vegetables to add flavor. Or use an edible oil spray to get a thin film. The plan includes fatty meats like nuts and pork. Add a light oil dressing to the salad. This means that you are more likely to ingest fat-soluble vitamins.

4. **Lemon or orange dressing acids are said to absorb more iron.** From lush greens such as spinach and kale. Watercress and orange are a great combination with a small number of sesame seeds and sunflower seeds or blanching almonds interspersed with a small amount of protein and crunch.

5. **Cook in a pan.** To reduce high-calorie fats. If the food sticks, splash the water.

6. **Weigh the food after cooking.** For an accurate calorie count.

7. **Dairy products are also included.** Choose low-fat cheese and skim milk, avoid high-fat yogurt, and choose a low-fat alternative. Drop the latte and throw the butter on a simple day. These are calorie traps.

8. **Similarly, avoid starchy white carbohydrates.** Avoid foods like bread, potatoes, or pasta and instead choose low GI carbohydrates such as vegetables, legumes, and slow-burning cereals. Choose brown rice and quinoa. Use oatmeal for breakfast longer than regular grains.

9. **Make sure your fast contains fiber.** Eat apples and pears, eat oats for breakfast, and add leafy vegetables.

10. **If possible, add flavors.** Chili flakes kick a delicious dish. Balsamic vinegar gave acidity. We also add fresh herbs—they are practically calorie-free but give the plate its personality.

11. **If you eat protein, you stay longer.** Stick to low-fat proteins, including some nuts and legumes. Remove meat skins and fats before cooking.

12. **Soup on a hungry day can be a savior.** Especially if you choose a light soup with leafy greens (Vietnamese Pho is ideal, but keeps the noodles low). Soup is a great way to consume the ingredients that you are fed up with and that you struggle with within the fridge.

13. **If desired, use agave as a sweetener. Lower GI.**

CHAPTER 9:

Common Mistakes

When it comes to intermittent fasting for beginners, it is necessary to avoid these misconceptions and mistakes no matter your age.

Rushing Into Intermittent Fasting

You are more likely to get hungry all the time and discouraged if you are regularly eating every 3–4 hours and then unexpectedly shrink your mealtime to only 8 hours. According to some experts, any individuals will stop intermittent fasting if they start by fasting for many hours without a transition time from a prior eating style. It can take between 10 days to 2 weeks for someone to quit feeling hungry when they fast. One of the greatest errors you can create is to start dramatically.

You can set yourself up for failure if you dive into IF without easing into it. It may be not easy to move from consuming 3 regular-sized meals or 6 tiny meals per day to eating only within 4 hours.

Instead, ease slowly into fasting. If you are going for the 16:8 technique, progressively increase the period between meals so you can operate inside 12 hours comfortably. Then, add multiple hours a day before you get to the 8-hour window.

There are levels of intermittent fasting. The primary factor most diets don't harvest benefits is their drastic deviation from our normal, usual eating habits. Sometimes, it can seem not easy to sustain. You think about it if someone is new to IF, then they are used to eating every 2 hours, you are going to very uncomfortable during long hours of fasting. It is normal to have a transition time, but it should feel better.

A remarkably strong communicator is the body itself. If it feels like trouble, it will let you know. And it is a common fact that you are going to feel like crap to starve yourself out of literally nowhere for 23 hours.

If you are stubborn about the principle of fasting, begin with the 12:12 approach of a beginner: fast for 12 hours a day and feed in the next 12-hour window.

That is pretty similar to what a person is used to doing nowadays, and who knows that it could be the only practical way to pursue it. You should level up to 16:8 once it seems comfortable, where you consume over an 8-hour window and fast during the remainder of the day. The best thing about IF is its simplicity, so choose a schedule that encourages you to adhere to a time frame without feeling bad. The number of hours one goes between meals is slowly extended until they hit a 12-hour feeding time. Then switch to an eating window of 10 hours and decrease by tiny amounts before meeting your target.

Expecting Intermittent Fasting to Change Your Life

Another error people seem to make is that they make their lives more about fasting than living. Because someone is fasting, they don't need to turn down the dinner request from their mates or a birthday celebration. That is not going to make it less satisfying and can still maintain such a lifestyle. Instead, on days where you have commitments with people, move your day backward or forward by a couple of hours so you can always enjoy socializing.

Choosing the Wrong Fasting Plan for Yourself

If you are trying something that would make your lifestyle difficult, it is not going to be the best option. Don't sign yourself up for disappointment, fasting only for few days then going back to your previous unhealthy ways will not be good for you. It is about adjusting the lifestyle you can maintain over a long time. Don't try to start the fast at 6 p.m. if someone is a night person. If someone is a regular gym-goer, then pick a fasting schedule that will suit your style.

Anyone else doesn't know your lifestyle. The specialist is you. And you have to make changes if you want to stick to the fasting pattern. If one is ready to pursue intermittent fasting and look for whole grains and healthy food such as fish, chicken and fruits, vegetables, and nutritious sides such as tofu, legumes, and quinoa for weight loss, then fasting will benefit you. The issue is, if you have not picked the right IF strategy, it will not give you success. Like if you are a committed gym-goer 6 days each week, the perfect schedule might not be to do fasting entirely on 2 of those days.

Not Drinking Enough and Drinking the Wrong Stuff

One intermittent fasting error to avoid is consuming the wrong drinks and not drinking sufficiently while fasting. Even if it is calorie-free, you don't want to consume something that is overly sweetened. Since it also has a detrimental impact on insulin levels and will stimulate your appetite and make you want to snack.

When fasting, aim to stick to water, pure tea, or black coffee. If one doesn't drink sufficiently, it may also cause dehydration, contributing to headaches, muscle cramps, and exacerbating hunger pangs.

Overeating When Fasting Ends

Overeating after completing the fast is another famous error. When a fast end, it may be simple to overeat simply because one may feel ravenous, or people justify themselves because they made up for missed calories, which is why they overeat.

But if you are fasting for weight reduction especially, this may turn out badly and even trigger some issues, including stomach aches. Prepare your meals beforehand; when your fast finishes, cook a nutritious recipe that is available for you and ensure that you consume whole foods wherever possible, including healthy carbohydrates such as seafood, vegetables, lean protein, and whole grains.

To avoid this, all you have to do is schedule your day, including the fasting and eating period ahead, ensuring that you eat healthy and keto-friendly foods after breaking the fast.

Eating Too Much in the Fasting Window

Most of the time, people want to pursue intermittent fasting because it involves eating fewer calories; it means they also will have less time to eat. In the duration of the fasting window, though, certain individuals will consume their normal amount of calories. This will imply you are not going to lose weight. Don't consume the normal intake of calories in the window. Rather, when one breaks the fast, expect to consume about 1,200–1,500 calories. If it is 4, 6, 8 hours, how many meals one can consume would depend on the duration of the fasting window.

If you need to overeat and are in a condition of starvation. Reconsider the strategy you want to adopt or relax off the IF for a day to regroup and then get back on board.

Forcing It on Your Self

Forcing the body to do fast another error. It is necessary to note that it is not for everybody to start intermittent fasting. It is all right to re-assess if this is the best strategy for you. Yes, some say that our bodies will cope quite frequently with hunger, but that doesn't imply that it is the best thing for everyone to do right now.

Not all bodies are developed for intermittent fasting. Ask yourself this easy question if intermittent fasting seems like a relentless challenge and emotional drain: Is the compromised standard of life worth it?

Not Paying Attention to the Nutrient Quality of the Foods

When following intermittent fasting, people often rely on fast foods when they simply concentrate on what to eat more than what they should consume. Instead of keeping a well-balanced diet, if you continue with refined foods, you should not anticipate intermittent fasting to achieve your fitness goals. By adopting nutritious foods steadily, aim to adjust your lifestyle along with your meal routine progressively.

Restricting the Food Intake Too Much

Not eating sufficient and going too far with fasting. You have got to note that fasting is not for starving. Our bodies need fuel to move around, work properly, think straight, and converse naturally, and that fuel comes from food. It takes a toll on daily life to limit your food consumption so much, and that is not the main concern of what fasting is all about.

The "what" is overlooked in favor of the "when." IF is a time-centered diet, and most schedules don't include any clear guidelines during the feeding window for the kinds of food to consume. Although this is not an accessible invitation for French fries, beer, and milkshakes, to thrive. Fasting is not magic. In addition to certain minor physiological effects, the main influence on weight reduction is that you minimize the hours of feeding and the number of calories you eat. If you have already had a pre-workout snack, it can sound alien to exercise when fasting. But when there are no calories, the body has loads of resources left in the body fat to use. As for every diet or workout schedule, consulting with the doctor first is a smart practice, but with intermittent fasting, exercising may be healthy.

Keep up with your normal fitness regimen or do something like cycling that is low-impact. You should consume a protein-rich meal after that. Always make sure to consult with your doctor first, as over 50 you should not do strenuous exercises while fasting.

Sadly, by selecting the wrong types of foods, you can't easily reverse the influence. During the feeding hours, change your mindset from a "treating yourself" attitude to one that centers on consuming the most nutrient-packed, nourishing meals you can find. To better fill yourself up and carry you during the fasting process, we suggest making sure any meal or snack contains a mix of fiber, protein, and good fats. Here are some tips that we provide for a better food intake:

- Cook all the meals at home and try not to eat takeout's or in restaurants.
- Pay attention to nutrition labels and make sure to not consume forbidden ingredients like modified palm oil, corn syrup, high fructose.
- Try to consume low sodium and beware of added sugar.
- Don't eat processed foods and home cook whole foods.
- Add fiber, good fats, and fiber to your plate, and lean proteins.

JUDITH E. KELLEY

CHAPTER 10:

Intermittent Fasting and Exercise

Women above 50 have a hard time taking care of their bodies if they are not active. Our body is unhealthy if it is subjected too long to a sedimentary lifestyle. There are multiple reasons for it. Some of the most active women I have seen in their 50s moved around their bodies quite a lot. They exercised their bodies, easily staying fit even when they aged. There were also the cases of women who were only 45 but they had the problems of 65 years older women. I expected as much seeing their sedimentary lifestyle. The exercise makes a hell lot of difference.

When you move around your body, you automatically push your body to regulate its functions, performing well. The body needs exercise just as our functions need to perform well. Exercise is the biggest difference-maker. It is that healthy habit that decides if you will automatically have a body of 30 years old while remaining 50 or have a body of 65 years old while remaining 40.

Generally, there are 2 kinds of females. The first type of females includes those ladies who have remained active in their youth. When they were in their 20s or 30s even, they moved around quite a lot. Yoga, jogging, and aerobics are something known to them. Naturally, they are also women who can do intermittent fasting better. Even if you are a woman in your 50s, you will remain much fitter if you exercised in your prime years.

There is another type of female who has led a sedimentary style of life. Those females are often inactive, lacking any interest in exercise or physical activity. Often, the busy routine along with a field of work makes this thing possible.

I can give you a piece of good news. Females who have not exercised in their 20s or even 30s can still reap the benefits of exercise. As you do intermittent fasting, you will realize that your bodies are more mobile than before, easily being able to do things you didn't think were possible. Even if you were a female who had led a life of physical inactiveness, you still have a shot at it. Intermittent fasting naturally reduces cholesterol, leading to a mobile and active body.

For the females who had been quite active before and still do a tremendous amount of exercise, I would suggest cutting down a bit. Intermittent fasting combined with exercise is somewhat a powerful combo for weight loss and cholesterol reduction. However, you must avoid exhaustion. I will give a list of the best exercises that are well suited for women above 50. You can choose a suitable time for these exercises like in the morning or evening. Make sure never to overexert your body. Your body is your temple and the more you take care of it, the more it will take care of you.

Walking/Jogging

This exercise is for females who have led an inactive lifestyle. You can start with 30 minutes, walk in the park or even your home. Gradually increase it to 45 minutes if possible. Walking is an amazing exercise if practiced daily. It is also the most basic form of exercise, leading females into a sense of activity. Interestingly, it is also preferred by women who were once very active but now have gone inactive physically. The best thing about walking is that it can be done on your own street or even rooftop.

An advanced form of walking is jogging. You can try it out in the park. When you start with walking and then gradually move towards jogging, there are a lot of benefits you will reap. Not only will your physical body be more active, but your mental health will also benefit from it.

Light Aerobics

You have not got much time? Or perhaps walking across the street or park is not possible? Light aerobics might just be what you need. You can start with light aerobics or low-impact aerobics. There are a lot of YouTube videos available online. You can take a start from there. You will only need to do these 20 minutes a day for 3–4 days per week. The best thing about aerobics is that it easily provides an amazing exercise in a very short time. It doesn't require any equipment. All you need is a laptop to watch its video from and an empty space like a room. Don't exert too much pressure on your body. The fellows in the videos are experts. You just have to do the exercise and move your body.

Stretching/Yoga

The stretching exercises are naturally the best ones. You can easily do yoga for adults on an everyday basis. The best results come when you pair it with light aerobics or walking. Yoga or stretching exercises have immense benefits. They relieve joint pain, provide your bones strength and flexibility and increase your immunity. The stretching exercises also allow your body to be more flexible and strong. Other than that, your mind will be relaxed as your body does the stretching.

Yoga poses for adult women are easily available online. The same rule with light aerobics goes here too. You will need to take it easy and slow. Only stretch your body till a mild discomfort. Don't push too hard.

Yoga routine is easily available. If you are someone who has not exercised for years, then yoga is for you too. Naturally, the best duo I have seen in some females was doing mild yoga in the morning and pairing it with light aerobics or walking in the evening.

In case if you do intermittent fasting, even simple yoga might be enough. Your body has already decreased the calorie intake and simple exercises will mold it into a perfect figure.

Balance

There are plenty of light exercises that focus on improving your balance. Naturally, some poses of yoga also focus on balance. It is somewhat a crucial part of your health. You should focus on it quite often.

JUDITH E. KELLEY

CHAPTER 11:

Breakfast

Healthy Chia and Oats Smoothie

Preparation time: 10 minutes
Cooking time: 0 minutes
Servings: 2
Ingredients

- 6 tbsp. oats
- 2 tbsp. chia seeds
- 2 tbsp. hemp powder
- 4 Medjool dates, pitted (optional)
- 2 bananas, chopped
- 1 c. almond milk
- 1 c. frozen berries
- 2 big handful's spinach, torn

Directions

1. Add all the ingredients to a blender and blend until smooth.
2. Pour in glasses and serve.

Nutrition

- Calories: 140 kcal.
- Fat: 7 g.
- Fiber: 4 g.
- Carbohydrates: 12 g.
- Protein: 12 g.

Cherry Almond and Cereal Smoothie

Preparation time: 10 minutes
Cooking time: 0 minutes
Servings: 2

Ingredients

- 1 c. fresh cherries, pitted + extra to garnish
- ¼ c. rolled oats
- 1 tbsp. hemp seeds
- 1 c. almond milk

Directions

1. Add all the ingredients to a blender and blend until smooth.
2. Pour into glasses and serve garnished with cherries.

Nutrition

- Calories: 200 kcal.
- Fat: 8 g.
- Fiber: 4 g.
- Carbohydrates: 8 g.
- Protein: 3 g.

Banana Orange Smoothie

Preparation time: 10 minutes
Cooking time: 0 minutes
Servings: 2
Ingredients

- 2 c. fat-free milk
- 1 c. nonfat Greek yogurt
- 1 medium banana
- 1 c. collard greens
- 1 orange, peeled, deseeded, separated into segments
- 6 strawberries, chopped
- 2 tbsp. sesame seeds

Directions

1. Add all the ingredients to a blender and blend until smooth.
2. Pour in glasses and serve.

Nutrition

- Calories: 183 kcal.
- Fat: 8 g.
- Fiber: 1 g.
- Carbohydrates: 3 g.
- Protein: 9 g.

Crunchy Banana Yoghurt

Preparation time: 10 minutes
Cooking time: 0 minutes
Servings: 4

Ingredients

- 3 c. fat-free natural Greek-style yogurt
- 1 oz. mixed seeds or nuts of your choice like pumpkin seeds, etc.
- 2 bananas, sliced

Directions

1. Take 4 bowls and add ¾ c. yogurt into each bowl.
2. Divide the banana slices among the bowl.
3. Sprinkle seeds on top and serve.

Nutrition

- Calories: 323 kcal.
- Fat: 11 g.
- Fiber: 4 g.
- Carbohydrates: 13 g.
- Protein: 17 g.

Grapefruit Yogurt Parfait

Preparation time: 10 minutes
Cooking time: 5 minutes
Servings: 4
Ingredients

- ½ c. amaranth
- 1 grapefruit, peeled, separated into segments, deseeded, and chopped
- 3 tbsp. toasted coconut
- Stevia to taste (optional)
- 1 c. plain, nonfat yogurt

Directions

1. Place a pan over medium heat. Add amaranth and let it pop. It should take 3–5 minutes. Let it cool for a few minutes.
2. Add yogurt into a bowl. Add Stevia and stir. Add 2 tbsp. yogurt into each of 4 glasses.
3. Place a layer of grapefruit in each glass. Add 1 tbsp. popped amaranth and sprinkle some coconut into the glasses.
4. Repeat steps 2–3 until all the ingredients are used up.

Nutrition

- Calories: 103 kcal.
- Fat: 4 g.
- Fiber: 1 g.
- Carbohydrates: 3 g.
- Protein: 22 g.

Creamy Mango and Banana Overnight Oats

Preparation time: 10 minutes
Cooking time: 0 minutes
Servings: 1
Ingredients
For the smoothie:

- 1 ripe banana
- ½ mango, peeled, cubed
- ½ tbsp. ground flaxseed
- 1 c. almond milk

For the oats:

- ⅓ c. oats
- 1 small ripe banana, mashed
- ½ c. almond milk
- ½ tbsp. ground flaxseed
- 2 tbsp. chia seeds
- Stevia or erythritol to taste

Directions

1. Add all the smoothie ingredients into a blender and blend until smooth.
2. Pour into a tall glass.
3. To make the oats layer: Add oats, almond milk, flaxseed, chia seeds, and stevia into a bowl. Stir well and add banana. Mix until well combined. Pour it over the smoothie in the glass.
4. Chill in the refrigerator overnight and serve.

Nutrition

- Calories: 199 kcal.
- Fat: 8 g.
- Fiber: 4 g.
- Carbohydrates: 9 g.
- Protein: 4 g.

Bacon and Eggs With Tomatoes

Preparation time: 10 minutes
Cooking time: 30 minutes
Servings: 5
Ingredients

- 4 large ripe tomatoes, halved
- 8 rashers smoked back bacon, trimmed of fat
- 4 eggs
- Salt to taste
- Pepper to taste
- 1 tsp. vinegar

Directions

1. Set up the grill to preheat. Let it preheat to high heat.
2. Place a rack on the grill pan. Line the pan with foil. Place tomatoes on the rack. Let it grill for 3 minutes. Place bacon along with the tomatoes.
3. Grill for 4 minutes until soft.
4. Meanwhile, place a large saucepan over medium-high heat. Fill the saucepan up to about ¾ with water. Let it boil.
5. When it begins to boil, add vinegar and stir. Crack 1 egg into a bowl and slowly slide the egg into the boiling water. Repeat this, one at a time.
6. Cook each egg until it is soft-boiled, for 2–3 minutes.
7. Meanwhile, divide the bacon and tomatoes into 2 plates.
8. Remove the eggs with a slotted spoon and place them on the plates. Sprinkle salt and pepper and serve.

Nutrition

- Calories: 110 kcal.
- Fat: 10 g.
- Fiber: 1 g.
- Carbohydrates: 3 g.
- Protein: 6 g.

Cinnamon Porridge

Preparation time: 10 minutes
Cooking time: 30 minutes
Servings: 4
Ingredients

- 4 ½ oz. jumbo porridge oats
- 20 oz. semi-skimmed milk
- 1 tsp. lemon juice
- ½ tsp. ground cinnamon + extra to garnish
- 2 ripe medium pears, peeled, cored, and grated

Directions

1. Add oats, milk, and cinnamon into a nonstick saucepan. Place the saucepan over medium-low heat. Cook until creamy. Stir constantly.
2. Divide into bowls. Scatter pear on top. Drizzle lemon juice on top. Garnish with cinnamon and serve.

Nutrition

- Calories: 383 kcal.
- Fat: 14 g.
- Fiber: 4 g.
- Carbohydrates: 3 g.
- Protein: 8 g.

CHAPTER 12:

Lunch

Lemon Baked Salmon

Preparation time: 5 minutes
Cooking time: 20 minutes
Servings: 2
Ingredients
- 12 oz. fillets of salmon
- 2 lemons, sliced thinly
- 2 tbsps. olive oil
- Salt and black pepper, to taste
- 3 sprigs thyme

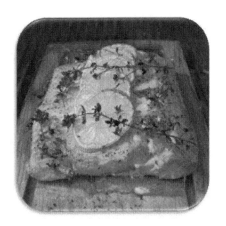

Directions
1. Preheat the oven to 350°F.
2. Place half the sliced lemons on the bottom of a baking dish.
3. Place the fillets over the lemons and cover with the remaining lemon slices and thyme.
4. Drizzle olive oil over the dish and cook for 20 minutes.
5. Season with salt and pepper.

Nutrition
- Calories: 571 kcal.
- Carbohydrates: 2 g.
- Fat: 44 g.
- Protein: 42 g.

Easy Blackened Shrimp

Preparation time: 10 minutes
Cooking time: 6 minutes
Servings: 2

Ingredients

- ½ lb. shrimp, peeled and deveined
- 2 tbsp. blackened seasoning
- 1 tsp. olive oil
- Juice of 1 lemon

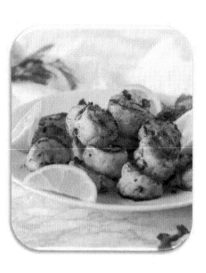

Directions

1. Toss all ingredients (except oil) together until shrimp are well coated.
2. In a nonstick skillet, heat the oil to medium-high heat.
3. Add shrimp and cook 2–3 minutes per side.
4. Serve immediately.

Nutrition

- Calories: 152 kcal.
- Carbohydrates: 5.1 g.
- Fat: 3.9 g.
- Protein: 24.4 g.

Grilled Shrimp Easy Seasoning

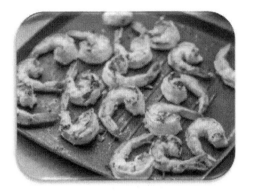

Preparation time: 5 minutes
Cooking time: 5 minutes
Servings: 4
Ingredients
For the shrimp seasoning:
- 1 tsp. garlic powder
- 1 tsp. kosher salt
- 1 tsp. Italian seasoning
- ¼ tsp. cayenne pepper

For the grilling:
- 2 tbsps. olive oil
- 1 tbsp. lemon juice
- 1 lb. jumbo shrimp, peeled, deveined
- Ghee for the grill

Directions
1. Preheat the grill pan to high.
2. In a mixing bowl, stir together the seasoning ingredients.
3. Drizzle in the lemon juice and olive oil and stir.
4. Add the shrimp and toss to coat.
5. Brush the grill pan with ghee.
6. Grill the shrimp until pink, about 2–3 minutes per side.
7. Serve immediately.

Nutrition
- Calories: 102 kcal.
- Carbohydrates: 1 g.
- Fat: 3 g.
- Protein: 28 g.

The Best Garlic Cilantro Salmon

Preparation time: 10 minutes
Cooking time: 15 minutes
Servings: 4

Ingredients

- 1 lb. salmon fillet
- 1 tbsp. butter
- 1 lemon
- ¼ c. fresh cilantro leaves, chopped
- 4 cloves garlic, minced
- ½ tsp. kosher salt
- ½ tsp. freshly cracked black pepper

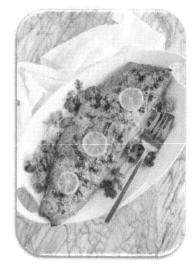

Directions

1. Preheat oven to 400°F.
2. On a foil-lined baking sheet, place salmon skin side down.
3. Squeeze lemon over the salmon.
4. Season salmon with cilantro, garlic, pepper, and salt.
5. Slice butter thinly and place pieces evenly over the salmon.
6. Bake for about 7 minutes, depending on thickness.
7. Turn the oven to broil and cook for 5–7 minutes, until the top is crispy.
8. Remove salmon from the oven and serve immediately.

Nutrition

- Calories: 140 kcal.
- Carbohydrates: 3.5 g.
- Fat: 4 g.
- Protein: 24.9 g.

Crispy Oven Roasted Salmon

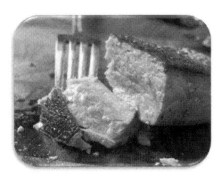

Preparation time: 5 minutes
Cooking time: 20 minutes
Servings: 3
Ingredients
- 1 lb. salmon fillet
- ¼ tsp. sea salt
- 2 tbsp. coconut oil
- ½ tsp. mixed herbs (oregano, thyme, marjoram)

Directions
1. Preheat the oven to 425°F.
2. Line a baking sheet with parchment paper and grease with 1 tbsp. of coconut oil.
3. Place the fillet on the lined baking sheet skin side down.
4. Season with salt and herbs.
5. Place 1 tbsp. of coconut oil on top of the salmon.
6. Cook for 20 minutes or until your desired level of crispiness is reached.
7. Serve immediately.

Notes: You can store the dish in a glass container in the fridge for up to 2 days.

Nutrition
- Calories: 400 kcal.
- Carbohydrates: 0.2 g.
- Fat: 28.7 g.
- Protein: 35.8 g.

Aromatic Dover Sole Fillets

Preparation time: 5 minutes
Cooking time: 20 minutes
Servings: 2

Ingredients

- 6 Dover Sole fillets
- ¼ c. virgin olive oil
- Zest of 1 lemon
- Dash of cardamom powder
- 1 c. fresh cilantro leaves
- Pinch of sea salt

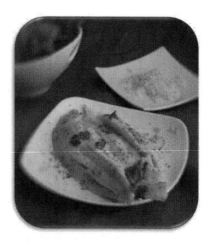

Directions

1. Bring the fillets to room temperature.
2. Set the oven's broiler to high.
3. Pour half of the oil into an oven tray.
4. Add half of the cilantro leaves, half of the lemon zest, and the cardamom powder.
5. Lay the fillets in the mixture and top with the remaining ingredients.
6. Set under the broiler for about 7–8 minutes or until the fish breaks easily with a fork and it is not transparent.
7. Serve immediately.

Nutrition

- Calories: 244 kcal.
- Carbohydrates: 2.9 g.
- Fat: 17.9 g.
- Protein: 18.6 g.

Bacon-Wrapped Salmon

Preparation time: 10 minutes
Cooking time: 20 minutes
Servings: 2
Ingredients

- 2 salmon fillets
- 1 tbsp. olive oil
- 4 slices bacon
- Lemon wedges
- 2 tbsp. tarragon

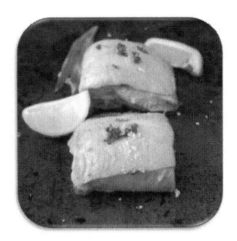

Directions
1. Preheat the oven to 350°F.
2. Pat the fillets dry.
3. Wrap bacon around the salmon fillets.
4. Place fillets on a roasting tray, and drizzle with olive oil.
5. Bake for 15–20 minutes.
6. Garnish with lemon wedges and chopped tarragon.

Nutrition

- Calories: 612 kcal.
- Carbohydrates: 7.1 g.
- Fat: 42 g.
- Protein: 53.3 g.

Japanese Fish Bone Broth

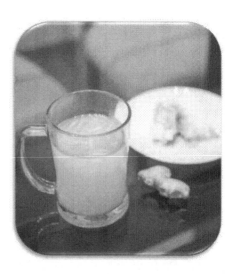

Preparation time: 5 minutes
Cooking time: 4 hours
Servings: 6–8

Ingredients
- Fish head and carcass
- 4 slices ginger
- 1 tbsp. lemon juice
- ½ leek, sliced
- Sea salt, to taste
- Water

Directions
1. Place the fish head and carcass into a large pot with cold water.
2. Bring to a boil and pour out the water.
3. Refill the pot with fresh water and add in the leek, sea salt, ginger, and lemon juice.
4. Simmer, covered, about 4 hours.

Nutrition
- Calories: 40 kcal.
- Carbohydrates: 0 g.
- Fat: 2 g.
- Protein: 5 g.

Ground Beef and Cauliflower Hash

Preparation time: 10 minutes
Cooking time: 25 minutes
Servings: 6
Ingredients

- 1 (16 oz.) bag of frozen cauliflower florets, defrosted and drained
- 1 lb. of lean grass-fed ground beef
- 2 c. of shredded Cheddar cheese
- 1 tsp. of garlic powder
- ½ tsp. of fine sea salt
- ½ tsp. of freshly cracked black pepper

Directions

1. In a large skillet over medium-high heat, add the ground beef and cook until brown. Drain the excess grease.
2. Add the cauliflower florets, garlic powder, fine sea salt, and freshly cracked black pepper. Cook until the cauliflower is tender, stirring occasionally.
3. Add the shredded Cheddar cheese to the cauliflower and ground beef mixture.
4. Remove from the heat and cover with a lid. Allow the steam to melt the cheese.
5. Serve and enjoy!

Nutrition

- Calories: 311 kcal.
- Fat: 7 g.
- Fiber: 2 g.
- Carbohydrates: 5 g.
- Protein: 33 g.

JUDITH E. KELLEY

CHAPTER 13:

Dinner

Garlic Ghee Pan-Fried Cod

Preparation time: 5 minutes
Cooking time: 10 minutes
Servings: 4
Ingredients
- 1 ¼ lb. cod fillets
- 3 tbsps. ghee
- 6 cloves of garlic, minced
- 1 tbsp. garlic powder
- A pinch salt

Directions
1. In a frying pan on medium-high heat, melt the ghee.
2. Add half the minced garlic.
3. Place the cod fillets in the pan and sprinkle with garlic powder and salt.
4. Cook until fish is a solid white color, about 4–5 minutes.
5. Then flip the fillets and add the remaining minced garlic. Cook until the whole fillets turn a solid white color, about 4–5 minutes.
6. Serve with the ghee and garlic from the pan.

Nutrition
- Calories: 160 kcal.
- Carbohydrates: 1 g.
- Fat: 7 g.
- Protein: 21 g.

Thyme Roasted Salmon

Preparation time: 10 minutes
Cooking time: 20 minutes
Servings: 4

Ingredients

- 1 lb. fresh salmon, skinless
- 2 tsp. olive oil
- ¼ tsp. kosher salt
- 1 tbsp. ghee
- ½ tsp. dried thyme
- Lemon wedges

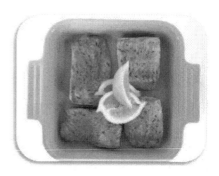

Directions

1. Preheat oven to 400°F.
2. Cut salmon into 4 equal-sized pieces.
3. Line a sheet pan with parchment paper and place salmon on it.
4. Brush with olive oil and season with salt.
5. Roast for 10 minutes.
6. In a small bowl, mix dried thyme and ghee. Set aside.
7. After 10 minutes of cooking, brush salmon with thyme-ghee mixture.
8. Roast for 5–8 minutes more, or until salmon is just cooked through.
9. Before serving, allow resting for 10 minutes.

Nutrition

- Calories: 186 kcal.
- Carbohydrates: 0 g.
- Fat: 9 g.
- Protein: 25 g.

Steam Your Own Lobster

Preparation time: 10 minutes
Cooking time: 10 minutes
Servings: 4
Ingredients
- 4 lobster tails
- 1 sprig parsley

Directions
1. If the lobster tails are frozen, defrost them.
2. Before cooking, make a long slit in the underbelly of the lobster.
3. Fill a pot halfway with water. Place a steamer basket inside.
4. Once the water is boiling, place the lobster tails onto the steamer attachment.
5. Let boil for 8–9 minutes for fresh lobster and 10 minutes for defrosted lobster.
6. Garnish with parsley.

Notes: If using fresh lobster, steam it for 8–9 minutes.

Nutrition
- Calories: 100 kcal.
- Carbohydrates: 0 g.
- Fat: 0 g.
- Protein: 24 g.

Bacon With Brussels Sprouts and Eggs

Preparation time: 20 minutes
Cooking time: 10 minutes
Servings: 4
Ingredients

- 6 eggs large
- 1 c. Trimmed and halved Brussels sprouts
- ¼ tsp. black pepper freshly ground
- 6 slices Bacon
- ¼ tsp. Salt
- 2 tbsp. Olive oil extra virgin
- 3 tbsp. Buffalo sauce
- ¼ tsp. Flakes of red pepper
- ½ tsp. Powder of garlic
- 1 tsp. Fresh chives chopped

Directions

1. Heat your oven in advance at 425°F.
2. Get a mixing container and in it mix the halved Brussels sprouts, powder of garlic, flakes of red pepper, bacon, buffalo sauce, and olive oil.
3. Add the black pepper that has been freshly ground and the salt to season the mix.
4. Get a large baking sheet and cover it with the mixture evenly.
5. Place the large baking sheet into the oven you heated in advance and let it bake for 15 minutes when the bacon will be crispy and the Brussels sprouts tender.
6. Take the sheet out and use a wooden spoon to make 6 holes in the baked mixture. Crack the eggs and pour in the holes you made using the wooden spoon and sprinkle a little black pepper that has been freshly ground and salt to season the eggs. Return the baking sheet into the oven and bake for 10 minutes until the eggs are done. Take the baking sheet out of the oven and sprinkle the fresh chives and buffalo sauce on top before serving.

Nutrition

- Calories: 100 kcal. Fat: 7 g. Fiber: 2 g. Carbohydrates: 8 g.
- Protein: 6 g.

Pan-Fried Tilapia

Preparation time: 10 minutes
Cooking time: 10 minutes
Servings: 4
Ingredients

- 2 tilapia fillets
- Salt, to taste
- 2 tbsps. coconut oil

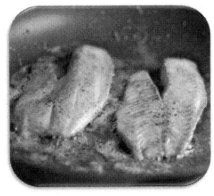

Directions
1. Add coconut oil to a frying pan on medium heat.
2. Salt the tilapia fillets.
3. Place the fillets in the frying pan and cook until fish is a solid white color, about 4–5 minutes. Then flip the fillets and cook until the whole fillets turn a solid white color, about 4–5 minutes.
4. Serve immediately.

Nutrition

- Calories: 91 kcal.
- Carbohydrates: 0.7 g.
- Fat: 1 g.
- Protein: 21 g.

Bacon Tacos

Preparation time: 10 minutes
Cooking time: 20 minutes
Servings: 4
Ingredients

- 14 pieces halved bacon - 1 avocado seeded, peeled, and sliced
- ¼ tsp. black pepper powder
- ½ c. Monterey Jack, shredded
- 5 eggs - 2 tbsp. fresh chives chopped
- 1 tbsp. almond milk - A pinch of salt
- 1 tbsp. unsweetened butter - A little hot sauce

Directions

1. Begin by preparing the taco shells first.
2. Heat the oven in advance at 400°F.
3. Get a baking sheet and line the inside with foil. Place the bacon strips in it, crisscrossing each other to form a square at the end. Do this again to form 3 consecutive weaves.
4. Take the black pepper powder and season the arranged bacon pieces and press flat the bacon using a baking rack that is inverted. Place the sheet for baking in the oven that you heated in advance and let the bacon bake until it is crispy, which will take 30 minutes. When the bacon is ready, using a knife for paring, cut up the crispy bacon squares to form small circles, which will be the taco shells. This should be done very fast.
5. Get the eggs and crack them in a mixing container. Add the almond milk and whisk both until they are well mixed.
6. Take a frying pan and over medium heat melt the unsweetened butter. Follow this by pouring the whisked egg mixture and slowly move the eggs around to turn them into scrambled eggs. Add salt and black pepper powder for seasoning followed by chives then remove the frying pan from the heat.
7. Get a plate that you will use to serve and arrange the bacon taco shells on top of it. Add the scrambled eggs on top of the bacon taco shells, then add a little cheese, avocado slices, and a little hot sauce as well.

Nutrition

- Calories: 260 kcal. Fat: 8 g. Fiber 2 g.
- Carbs 8 g. Protein: 45 g.

Calamari Rings

Preparation time: 5 minutes
Cooking time: 2 minutes
Servings: 4
Ingredients

- 4 calamari squid tubes
- 1 tbsp. ghee
- 2 tbsp. almond flour
- Zest and juice of 1 lemon
- Salt and pepper, to taste

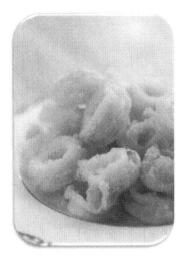

Directions
1. Mix the almond flour, lemon zest, salt, and pepper.
2. Slice the squid tubes into ½-inch slices.
3. Roll the calamari rings in the almond mix.
4. Heat ghee in a frying pan and fry rings on low heat for 1 minute on each side until cooked and golden.
5. Drizzle with lemon juice.

Nutrition

- Calories: 159 kcal.
- Carbohydrates: 5.9 g.
- Fat: 8.2 g.
- Protein: 16.3 g.

Pinchos de Pollo— Marinated Grilled Chicken Kebabs

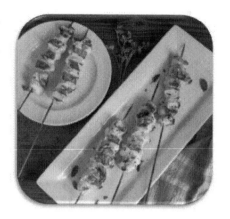

Preparation time: 10 minutes (+2 hours)
Cooking time: 10 minutes
Servings: 4
Ingredients

- 1 ½ lb. boneless, skinless chicken breast
- 1 tbsp. minced garlic
- ½ tsp. fine Himalayan salt
- ½ tsp. freshly ground black pepper
- 1 tsp. dried oregano
- 1 tbsp. extra-virgin olive oil
- Juice of 1 lime
- 7–9 skewers

Directions

1. Have ready 7–9 soaked skewers.
2. In a bowl, combine the salt, garlic, pepper, lime juice, oregano, and oil.
3. Cut chicken breast into 1-inch chunks and place in a container with a lid.
4. Pour the marinade over the chicken and stir. Cover and refrigerate at least for 2 hours or overnight.
5. Preheat a grill to 325–375°F.
6. Remove the chicken from the refrigerator and thread it onto the skewers, leaving a very small space between each piece and spreading each piece as flat as possible.
7. Once the grill is hot, grill the kebabs over direct medium heat, about 8–10 minutes total, keeping the lid closed until the chicken is no longer pink in the center and firm to the touch, turning once or twice during cooking. Take care not to overcook. Remove from the grill and serve immediately!

Nutrition

- Calories: 290 kcal. Carbohydrates: 3 g. Fat: 10 g.
- Protein: 9 g.

CHAPTER 14:

Snacks

Blueberries Bowl

Preparation time: 35 minutes
Cooking time: 0 minutes
Servings: 1
Ingredients

- 1 tsp. chia seeds
- 1 c. almond milk
- ¼ c. fresh blueberries or fresh fruits
- 1 pack sweetener for taste

Directions

1. Mix the chia seeds with almond milk. Stir periodically.
2. Place in the fridge to cool for 30 minutes, and then serve with fresh fruit. Enjoy!

Nutrition

- Calories: 202 kcal.
- Fat: 16.8 g.
- Protein: 10.2 g.
- Total carbohydrates: 9.8 g.
- Dietary fiber: 5.8 g.
- Net carbohydrates: 2.6 g.

Bacon and Chicken Garlic Wrap

Preparation time: 15 minutes
Cooking time: 10 minutes
Servings: 4

Ingredients

- 1 chicken fillet, cut into small cubes
- 8–9 thin slices bacon, cut to fit cubes
- 6 garlic cloves, minced

Directions

1. Preheat your oven to 400°F.
2. Line a baking tray with aluminum foil.
3. Add minced garlic to a bowl and rub each chicken piece with it.
4. Wrap bacon piece around each garlic chicken bite.
5. Secure with a toothpick.
6. Transfer bites to the baking sheet, keeping a little bit of space between them.
7. Bake for about 15–20 minutes until crispy.
8. Serve and enjoy!

Nutrition

- Calories: 260 kcal.
- Fat: 19 g.
- Carbohydrates: 5 g.
- Protein: 22 g.

Coated Cauliflower Head

Preparation time: 10 minutes
Cooking time: 40 minutes
Servings: 6
Ingredients

- 2 lb. cauliflower head
- 3 tbsps. olive oil
- 1 tbsp. butter, softened
- 1 tsp. ground coriander
- 1 tsp. salt
- 1 egg, whisked
- 1 tsp. dried cilantro
- 1 tsp. dried oregano
- 1 tsp. tahini paste

Directions

1. Trim cauliflower head if needed.
2. Preheat oven to 350°F.
3. In the mixing bowl, mix up together olive oil, softened butter, ground coriander, salt, whisked egg, dried cilantro, dried oregano, and tahini paste.
4. Then brush the cauliflower head with this mixture generously and transfer it to the tray.
5. Bake the cauliflower head for 40 minutes.
6. Brush it with the remaining oil mixture every 10 minutes.

Nutrition

- Calories: 136 kcal.
- Protein: 4.43 g.
- Fat: 10.71 g.
- Carbohydrates: 7.8 g.

Cauliflower Crust Pizza

Preparation time: 20 minutes
Cooking time: 42 minutes
Servings: 2
Ingredients
For the crust:

- 1 small head cauliflower, cut into florets
- 2 large organic eggs, beaten lightly
- ½ tsp. dried oregano
- ½ tsp. garlic powder
- Ground black pepper, as required

For the topping:

- ½ c. sugar-free pizza sauce
- ¾ c. Mozzarella cheese, shredded
- ¼ c. black olives, pitted and sliced
- 2 tbsps. Parmesan cheese, grated

Directions

1. Preheat your oven to 400°F (200°C). Line a baking sheet with lightly greased parchment paper.
2. Add the cauliflower to a food processor and pulse until a rice-like texture is achieved. In a bowl, add the cauliflower rice, eggs, oregano, garlic powder, and black pepper and mix until well combined. Place the cauliflower mixture in the center of the prepared baking sheet and with a spatula, press into a 13-inch thin circle. Bake for 40 minutes or until golden brown. Remove the baking sheet from the oven. Now, set the oven to broiler on high.
3. Place the pizza sauce on top of the pizza crust and with a spatula, spread evenly, and sprinkle with olives, followed by the cheeses. Broil for about 1–2 minutes or until the cheese is bubbly and browned. Remove from oven and with a pizza cutter, cut the pizza into equal-sized triangles.
4. Serve hot.

Nutrition

- Calories: 119 kcal. Fat: 6.6 g. Saturated fat: 1.8 g.
- Cholesterol: 98 mg. Sodium: 297 mg. Carbohydrates: 8.6 g.
- Fiber: 3.4 g. Sugar: 3.7 g. Protein: 8.3 g.

Cabbage Casserole
Preparation time: 15 minutes
Cooking time: 30 minutes
Servings: 2
Ingredients
- ½ head cabbage
- 2 scallions, chopped
- 4 tbsps. unsalted butter
- 2 oz. cream cheese, softened
- ¼ c. Parmesan cheese, grated
- ¼ c. fresh cream
- ½ tsp. Dijon mustard
- 2 tbsps. fresh parsley, chopped
- Salt and ground black pepper, as required

Directions
1. Preheat your oven to 350°F (180°C).
2. Cut the cabbage head into half, lengthwise. Then cut into 4 equal-sized wedges.
3. In a pan of boiling water, add cabbage wedges and cook, covered for about 5 minutes.
4. Drain well and arrange cabbage wedges into a small baking dish.
5. In a small pan, melt butter and sauté scallions for about 5 minutes.
6. Add the remaining ingredients and stir to combine.
7. Remove from the heat and immediately, place the cheese mixture over cabbage wedges evenly.
8. Bake for about 20 minutes.
9. Remove from the oven and let it cool for about 5 minutes before serving.
10. Cut into 3 equal-sized portions and serve.

Nutrition
- Calories: 273 kcal. Fat: 24.8 g.
- Saturated fat: 15.4 g. Cholesterol: 71 mg.
- Sodium: 313 mg. Carbohydrates: 9 g.
- Fiber: 3.4 g. Sugar: 4.5 g. Protein: 6.2 g.

Salmon With Salsa

Preparation time: 15 minutes
Cooking time: 8 minutes
Servings: 2
Ingredients
For the salsa:

- 1 small tomato, chopped
- 2 tbsps. red onion, chopped finely
- ¼ c. fresh cilantro, chopped finely
- 1 tbsp. jalapeño pepper, seeded and minced finely
- 1 garlic clove, minced finely
- Salt and ground black pepper, as required

For the salmon:

- 4 (5 oz.) (1-inch thick) salmon fillets
- 3 tbsps. butter
- 1 tbsp. fresh rosemary leaves, chopped
- 1 tbsp. fresh lemon juice
- Salt and ground black pepper, as required

Directions

1. **For the salsa:** Add all ingredients in a bowl and gently, stir to combine. With plastic wrap, cover the bowl and refrigerate before serving.
2. **For the salmon:** Season each salmon fillet with salt and black pepper generously. In a large skillet, melt butter over medium-high. Place the salmon fillets, skins side up, and cook for about 4 minutes. Carefully change the side of each salmon fillet and cook for about 4 minutes more. Stir in the rosemary and lemon juice and remove from the heat. Divide the salsa onto serving plates evenly. Top each plate with 1 salmon fillet and serve.

Nutrition

- Calories: 481 kcal. Fat: 37.2 g.
- Saturated fat: 10.9 g. Cholesterol: 85 mg.
- Sodium: 172 mg. Carbohydrates: 11 g.
- Fiber: 7.6 g. Sugar: 1.5 g. Protein: 29.9 g.

Artichoke Petals Bites

Preparation time: 10 minutes
Cooking time: 10 minutes
Servings: 8
Ingredients

- 8 oz. artichoke petals, boiled, drained, and without salt
- ½ c. almond flour
- 4 oz. Parmesan, grated
- 2 tbsps. almond butter, melted

Directions

1. In the mixing bowl, mix up together almond flour and grated Parmesan.
2. Preheat the oven to 355°F.
3. Dip the artichoke petals in the almond butter and then coat in the almond flour mixture.
4. Place them in the tray.
5. Transfer the tray to the preheated oven and cook the petals for 10 minutes.
6. Chill the cooked petal bites a little before serving.

Nutrition

- Calories: 93 kcal.
- Protein: 6.54 g.
- Fat: 3.72 g.
- Carbohydrates: 9.08 g.

JUDITH E. KELLEY

Conclusion

Thank you for making it to the end. As we end this book, here are some tips that you can use in order to make intermittent fasting successful and easier. You can start by skipping breakfast or giving up dinner if you really want to go all-in, but we recommend starting with the 16:8 method, which is skipping breakfast and lunch every day of the week or even adding another meal like dinner.

You should be able to overcome hunger. If you feel that you can't do it, then don't force it. Maybe you didn't try the 16:8 and are still eating 3 meals per day.

Drink lots of water, juice, and smoothies and eat vegetables to keep you hydrated and energized throughout the day. Remember, you are reducing the amount of food you eat, so you should also reduce the number of drinks and foodstuffs that contain calories.

Don't skip meals completely. If you can't do it by skipping meals entirely (like fasting for a few hours), there are plenty of other options like:

- **Intermittent fasting for a few hours:** For example, going to bed at 8 p.m. and waking up at 6 a.m. the next day is a short 16-hour fast. You could break up this fast with a 3-hour lunch break or dinner time meal.
- **Intermittent fasting for one meal per day:** In this case, the main meal will be skipped or eaten late in the evening when it contains mostly fat.
- **Intermittent fasting for several meals per day:** When you feel hungry, just have a small snack and wait until hunger subsides.

It is important to be consistent. If you stop fasting too often, especially for no reason at all, you will give up, and intermittent fasting will become something less than a diet.

You can fast for a long time if you really want to (if that is the case, it should be called "Fat Burning"), but don't go longer than 21–23 hours without eating anything or mix it with one of the other fasts (e.g., 16:8).

Don't use fasting as a tool for losing weight! If you do it the wrong way or are not physically active, this alone will lead to unnecessary weight loss, which is definitely not what we want!

Drink green tea during the fasting period or after your fasted period is over for extra energy boost and better health overall.

Avoid eating after 11 p.m. Eat, but only 5–6 hours before bedtime as this is enough time to let the body rest (some experts say 8 hours or more).

Even if you can eat whatever you want during the day, still drink lots of water and be aware of your food intake so that you don't gain too much weight.

If you can't stay with 16:8 yet, then instead of skipping breakfast and lunch every day, try to skip 4 meals a week or even 3 meals if you really need it! And also, avoid snacking between meals too much as many people tend to do it anyway.

Try to go to bed and wake up at the same time every day. This habit alone will make you feel better as your body will get used to it.

If you have never tried intermittent fasting before, then start with 16:8 (skipping breakfast and lunch every day of the week) and gradually add more meals or days to it.

I hope you have learned something!

Manufactured by Amazon.ca
Bolton, ON